Contents

Edition 12.2

Important

This book has been designed as a learning guide to a full first aid course and cannot replace hands on training in the skills of dealing with an emergency situation.

The circumstances in which illness and injury occur vary considerably and are outside the control of the author, so it is not possible to give definitive guidance for every situation. If you suspect illness or injury therefore, you should always seek immediate professional medical advice.

Whilst every effort has been made to ensure the accuracy of the information contained within this book, the author does not accept any liability for any inaccuracies or for any subsequent mistreatment, however caused.

Tel. 0845 644 3305 www.qualsafe.com

Introduction

This book has been written by an experienced paramedic, trainer and leading first aid author. It is designed specifically to guide you through your first aid course and to provide you with a quick reference guide for future years.

This book is fully compliant with UK and European Resuscitation and First Aid Guidelines.

Effective emergency treatment before professional help arrives can go a long way to reducing the effects of illness and injury and indeed save someone's life. Taking part in a first aid course and using this book may be the most important decision you make in your life...

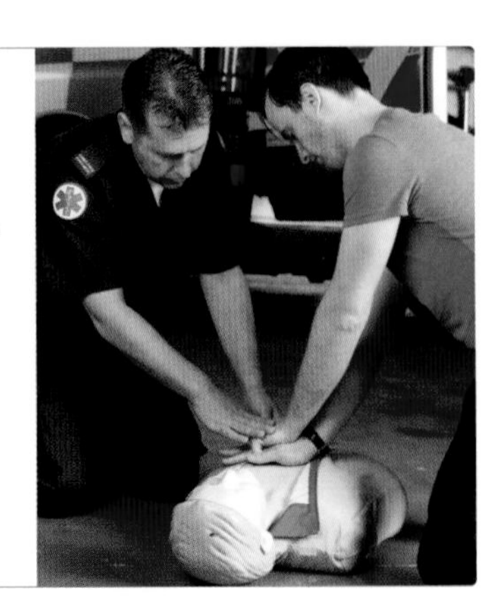

Clinical review panel

The accuracy of this book is reviewed and supported by a distinguished panel of experts in emergency medical care:

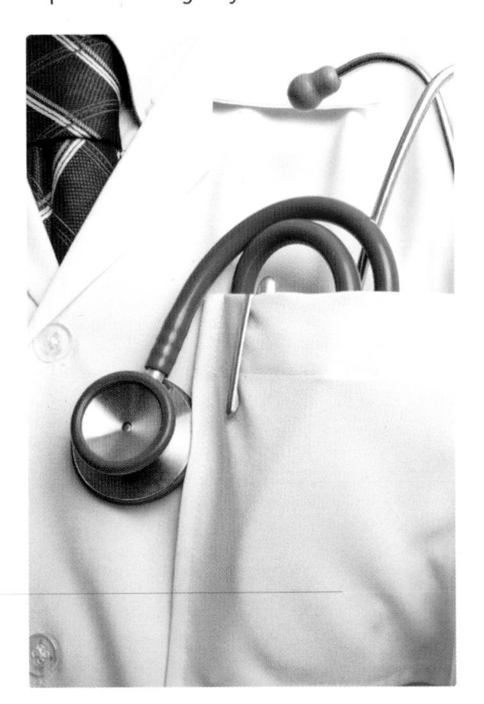

Professor Sir Keith Porter
Professor of Clinical Traumatology, Faculty of Pre-hospital Care Royal College of Surgeons *(Edinburgh)* Past President, citizenAID Co-founder.

Professor Andrew Lockey
Consultant in Emergency Medicine, President Resuscitation Council *(UK)*, ILCOR Education Group Member, Associate Dean Health Education England.

Doctor Rachel Oaten
Consultant in Emergency Medicine, Deputy Clinical Director Acute Medicine, Deputy Medical Director East Midlands Ambulance Service *(with clinical governance portfolio to Police and Fire)*, Wiltshire Police Clinical Governance Lead.

Doctor Sal Uka
Consultant Paediatrician, Fellow of the Royal College of Paediatrics and Child Health, Member of the British Paediatric Neurology Association.

Paramedic Nigel Barraclough
HCPC Registered Paramedic, Resuscitation Council UK Community & Ambulance Resuscitation Committee, First Aid Quality Partnership, Vice Chair First Aid Awarding Organisation Forum, Trustee citizenAID Charity.

The role of the first aider

First aid is defined as the 'help given to a sick or injured person until full medical treatment is available'. The Health and Safety *(First-Aid)* Regulations 1981 require an employer to provide suitable first aid cover in the workplace.

The responsibilities of a first aider include:

Assessing the situation

- Work out what has happened
- Count the number of casualties
- Look for history, signs and symptoms

Protecting from danger

- Assess for further dangers
- Protect yourself first, then protect others

Getting help

- Ask bystanders for assistance
- Work out what help is needed
- Call for help *(or ask a bystander to call)*
- Recognise your own limitations

Prioritising treatment

- Treat the most urgent thing first
- Treat the most urgent person first
- Offer support and comfort

Minimising infection risks

- Wear personal protective equipment *(PPE)* when needed *(especially during a disease outbreak such as COVID-19)*
- Casualty to wear a face mask if appropriate
- Wash hands before and after giving help
- Cover your own cuts with a plaster
- Dispose of contaminated waste carefully
- Use sterile, undamaged, in-date dressings

Consent

It is important to ask for the casualty's consent before giving first aid. Just touching someone without their permission could be classed as assault.

The law allows the assumption that an unconscious casualty gives consent.

The aims of first aid

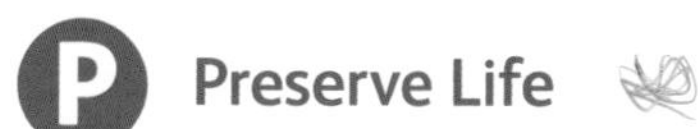

P Preserve Life 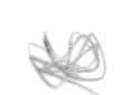

P Prevent the situation worsening 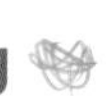

P Promote Recovery 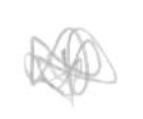

Personal protective equipment *(PPE)*

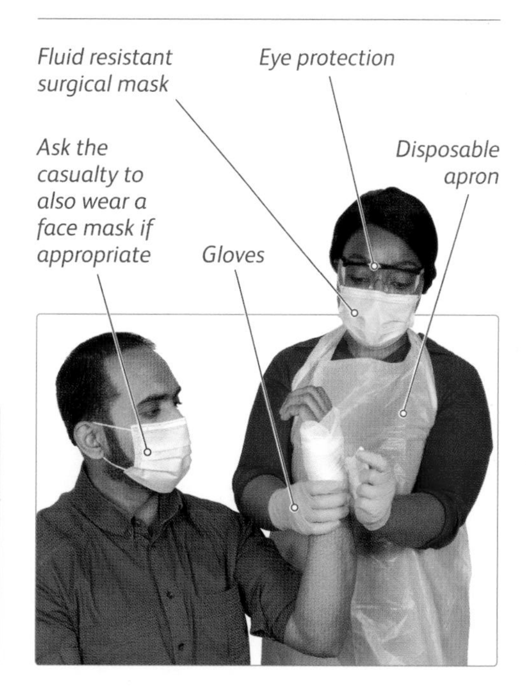

First aid kits

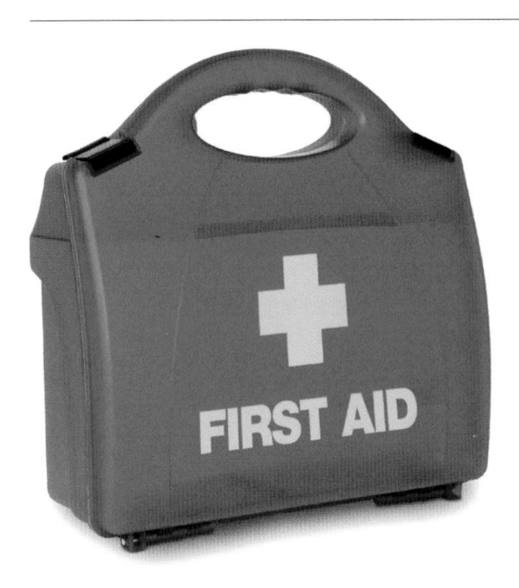

First aid kits should be identified by a white cross on a green background.

Most workplace first aid kits conform to British Standard BS 8599 and are available in different sizes to suit the environment.

If there is no mains tap water, have at least 1 litre of sterile water available for eye-washing.

PPE

Disposable gloves, aprons, face masks and eye protection should be available in or near a first aid kit *(see page 3)*.

NOTE: Tablets and medicines should not be stored in a first aid kit, because first aiders are not trained to administer or dispense them.

First aid equipment

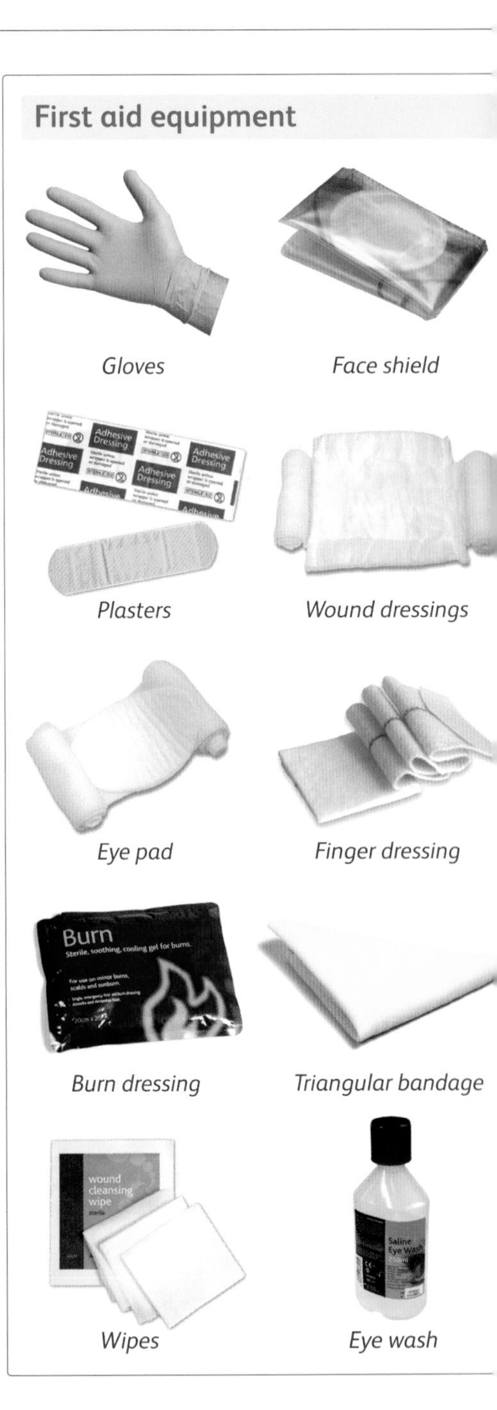

Gloves

Face shield

Plasters

Wound dressings

Eye pad

Finger dressing

Burn dressing

Triangular bandage

Wipes

Eye wash

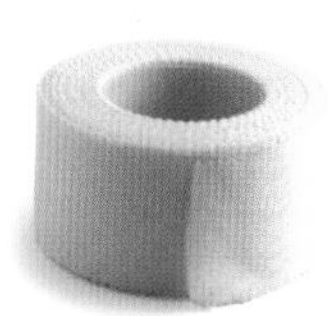
Adhesive tape

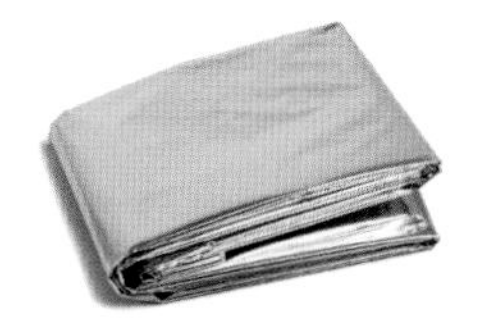
Foil blanket

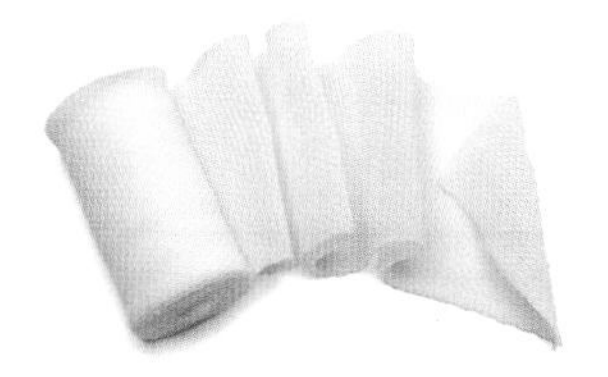
Conforming bandage

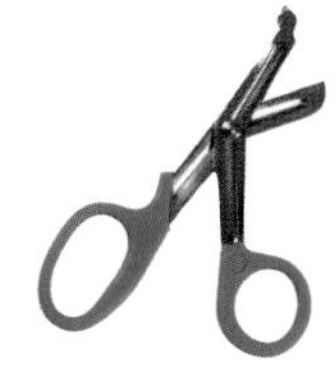
Shears

BS 8599-1:2019 workplace first aid kits

Recommended size of kit:	Small	Medium	Large	Travel	Personal	Critical injury
Lower Risk: e.g. Offices, shops and libraries etc.	Less than 25 employees	25 – 100 employees	More than 100 employees	For travel and motoring	For personal issue	For catastrophic bleeding control
Higher Risk: e.g. Food processing, assembly work, warehousing, engineering, construction, manufacturing etc.	Less than 5 employees	5 – 25 employees	More than 25 employees			

Contents:	Small	Medium	Large	Travel	Personal	Critical injury
Bandage, conforming	1	2	2	-	-	-
Bandage, triangular	2	3	4	1	1	-
Dressing pad, adhesive	-	-	-	1	-	-
Dressing, burn	1	2	2	2	-	-
Dressing, eye pad	2	3	4	-	-	-
Dressing, finger	2	3	4	-	-	-
Dressing, haemostatic	-	-	-	-	-	2
Dressing, sterile, large	2	3	4	-	1	-
Dressing, sterile, medium	2	4	6	1	-	-
Dressing, trauma, large	-	-	-	-	-	2
Dressing, trauma, medium	-	-	-	1	-	-
Foil blanket	1	2	3	1	1	1
Gloves, nitrile *(pairs)*	6	9	12	2	2	2
Guidance leaflet	1	1	1	1	1	1
Plasters, wash-proof	40	60	100	10	10	-
Resuscitation face shield	1	1	2	1	1	-
Shears *(for cutting clothing & leather)*	1	1	1	1	1	1
Tape, microporous	1	2	3	-	-	-
Tourniquet	-	-	-	-	-	1
Wipes, alcohol free	20	30	40	10	4	-

Accident recording

Any accident at work must be recorded. An accident report can be completed by the casualty, but often the first aider helps with this task.

The information recorded can help an employer to identify accident trends and possible areas of health and safety improvements. It can be used for future first aid needs assessments and may be helpful for insurance investigations.

The report should include:

- The name, address and occupation of the person who had the accident.
- The name, address, occupation and signature of the person who is completing the report.
- The date, time and location of the accident.
- A description of how the accident happened, giving the cause if you can.
- Details of the injury suffered.

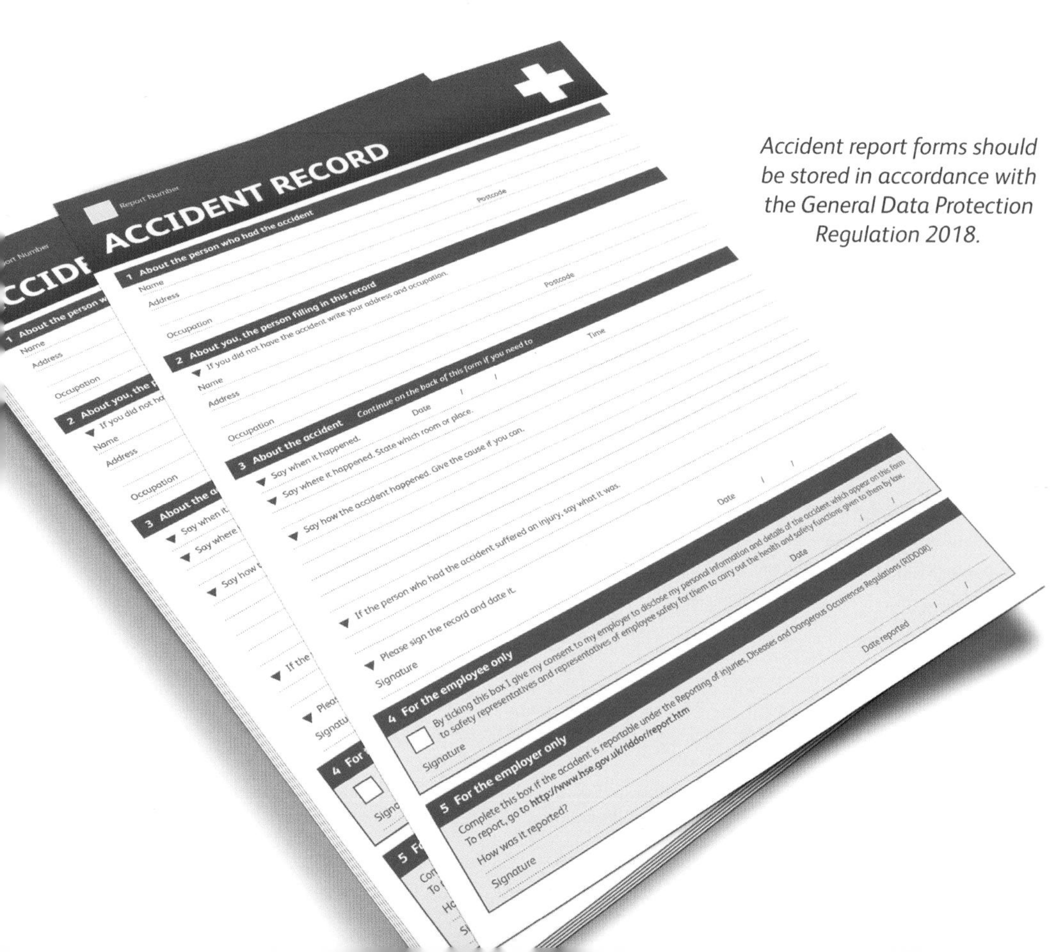

Report Number

ACCIDENT RECORD

1 About the person who had the accident

Name

Address

Postcode

Occupation

2 About you, the person filling in this record

▼ If you did not have the accident write your address and occupation.

Name

Address

Postcode

Occupation

3 About the accident Continue on the back of this form if you need to

▼ Say when it happened. Date / / Time

▼ Say where it happened. State which room or place.

▼ Say how the accident happened. Give the cause if you can.

▼ If the person who had the accident suffered an injury, say what it was.

▼ Please sign the record and date it.

Signature Date / /

4 For the employee only

By ticking this box I give my consent to my employer to disclose my personal information and details of the accident which appear on this form to safety representatives and representatives of employee safety for them to carry out the health and safety functions given to them by law.

Signature Date / /

5 For the employer only

Complete this box if the accident is reportable under the Reporting of Injuries, Diseases and Dangerous Occurrences Regulations (RIDDOR).

To report, go to **http://www.hse.gov.uk/riddor/report.htm**

How was it reported? Date reported / /

Signature

Accident report forms should be stored in accordance with the General Data Protection Regulation 2018.

Surveying the scene

Let's explore this scenario; there has been a serious accident at work.

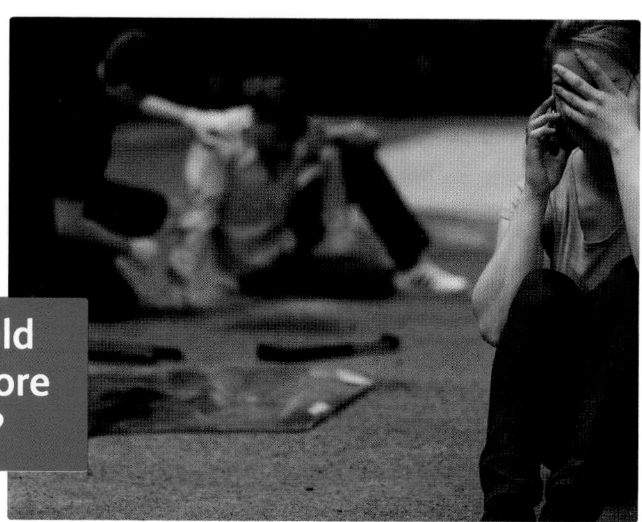

What things should you consider before treating anyone?

What happened?

- Working this out could answer some of the following questions...

Further danger?

- Can it happen again?
- Is there a risk of fire, explosion, collapse, chemicals, traffic, electricity, gas, drowning etc.?

Can you cope?

- Ask bystanders to help.
- Use others to make the scene safe *(e.g. traffic control at road incidents)*.
- Avoid individual tasks. Take charge and give jobs to others instead.

Number of casualties?

- This information is vital for emergency services.
- How many appear seriously injured?

Emergency services?

- What is the exact location?
- Fire and rescue?
- Ambulance?
- Police?

Who needs help first?

- Assess casualties using the 'Primary Survey' *(pages 8–9)*.
- If there are multiple casualties – tell others what to do.

Prioritising treatment – the primary survey

We need a constant supply of oxygen to survive. If our brain cells don't get oxygen, they start to die within 3 to 4 minutes.

The priorities of treatment are making sure oxygen gets into the blood and that the blood carries it to the brain.

The primary survey is a fast and systematic way to find and treat **life-threatening conditions** in priority order.

If a life-threatening condition is found, it should be treated **immediately**, before moving on to the next step.

Use DRABC *('Doctor ABC')* to remember the primary survey sequence.

"Perform a primary survey first on every casualty and until it's complete, do not be distracted by more superficial, non life-threatening conditions."

D

Danger

- Make sure you, the casualty and any bystanders are safe.
- Don't put your own life at risk – one casualty is enough!

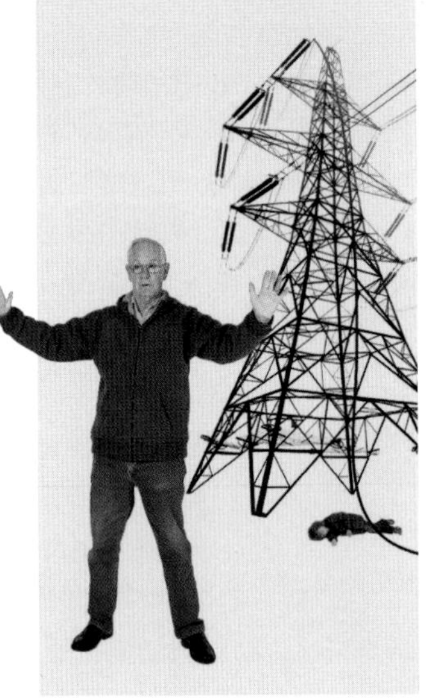

R

Response

- Quickly check to see if the casualty is conscious. Gently shake or tap the shoulders and ask loudly 'are you alright?'
- Unconscious casualties take priority and need urgent treatment.
- If an unconscious casualty is on their back, the **airway** can be at risk.

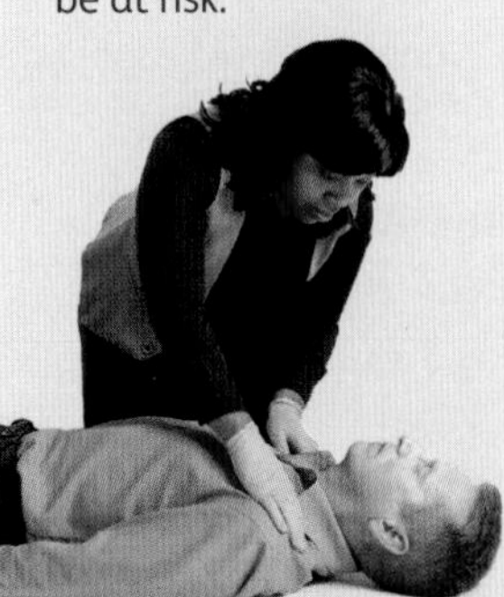

Multiple casualties

Use the DRABC primary survey to decide who needs treatment first. A rough rule of thumb is that the casualty who is the quietest needs treatment first, whereas the one making the most noise (trying to get your attention) is the least serious!

A

Airway

- Identify and treat any life-threatening **airway** problems *(see below)*.
- If the casualty is unconscious, tilt the head back to open the airway *(beware of neck injury – page 40)*.
- When the airway is clear/opened, move on to **Breathing**.

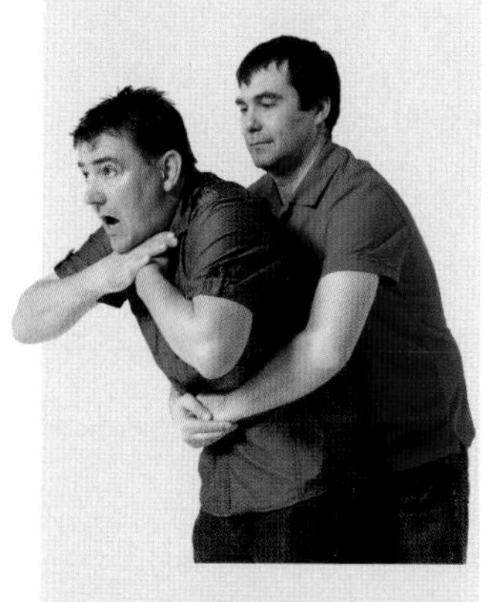

Life-threatening conditions:

Airway swelling, narrowing or blockage caused by:

The tongue, vomit, choking, burns, strangulation, hanging, anaphylaxis.

B

Breathing

- Identify and treat any life-threatening **breathing** problems *(see below)*.
- If the casualty is unconscious and not breathing normally, perform CPR *(page 10)*.
- When life-threatening breathing problems have been ruled out or treated, move on to **Circulation**.

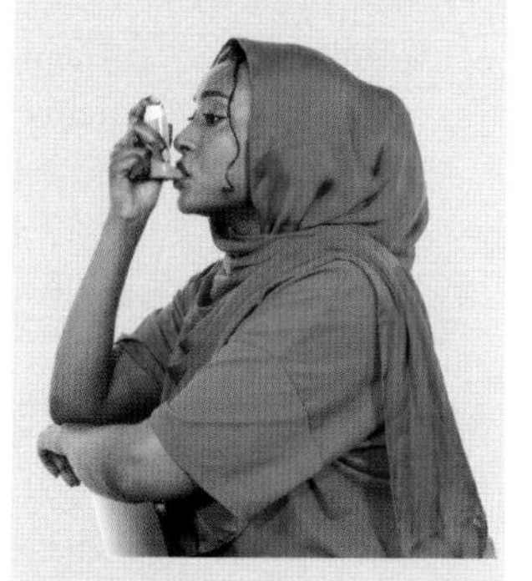

Life-threatening conditions:

Asthma, crushing of the chest, chest injury, collapsed lung, poisoning, anaphylaxis, cardiac arrest.

C

Circulation

- Identify and treat any life-threatening **circulation** problems *(see below)*.
- When life-threatening circulation problems have been ruled out or treated, the primary survey is complete. You can now perform a **Secondary survey** *(page 31)* to look for other conditions *(such as broken bones)*.

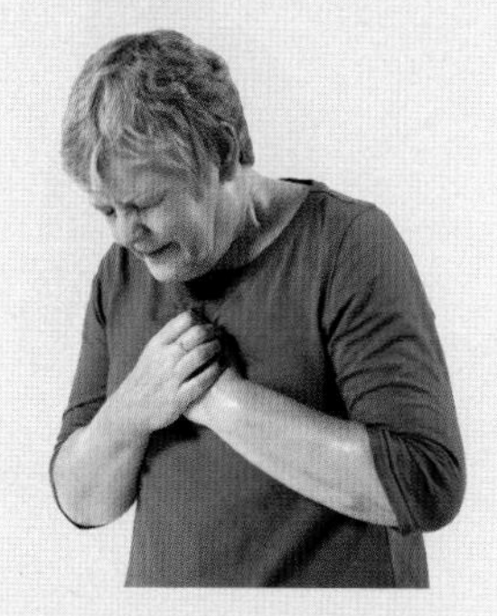

Life-threatening conditions:

Heart attack, heart failure, severe bleeding, poisoning, anaphylaxis, cardiac arrest.

Resuscitation *(CPR)*

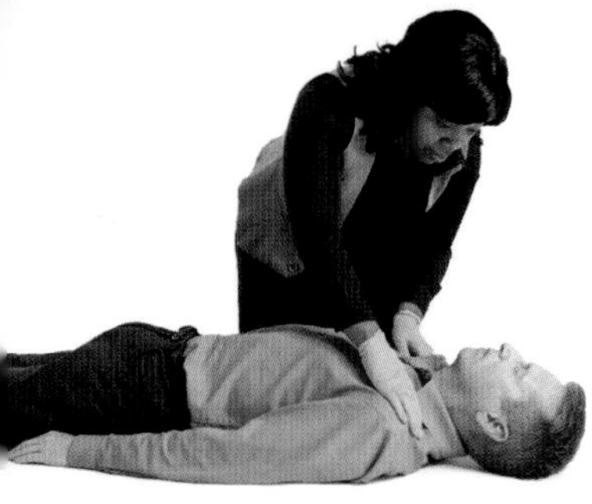

Gently shake the shoulders.

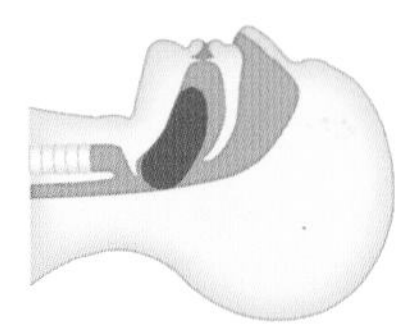

Airway blocked by the tongue.

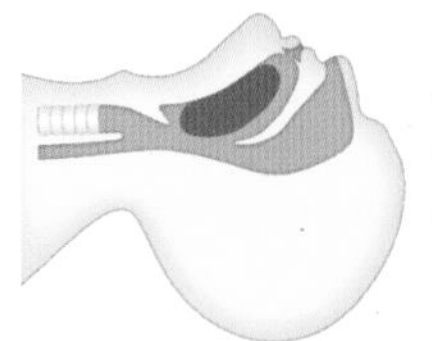

Airway cleared by tilting the head.

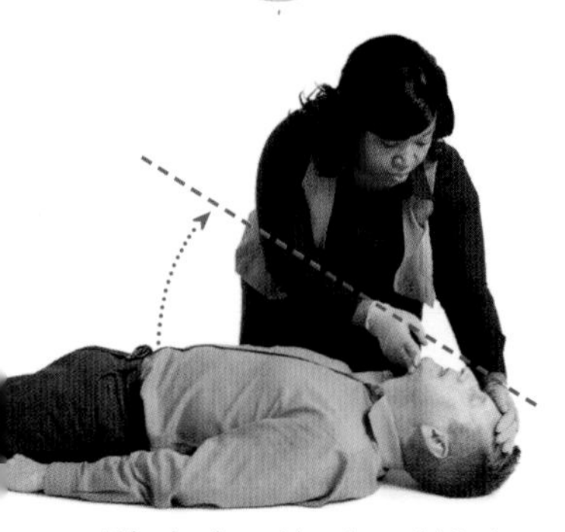

Tilt the head back and lift the chin to open the airway.

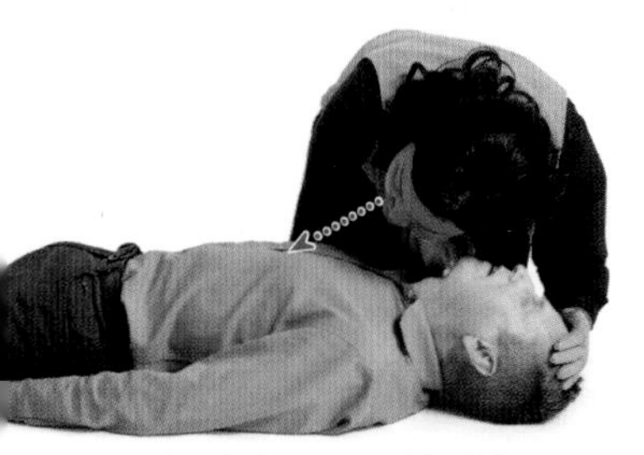

Look, listen and feel for normal breathing.

COVID-19 CPR – see page 64

Danger

- Make sure that you, the casualty and any bystanders are safe.

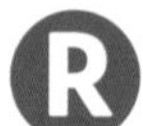

Response

- Gently shake the shoulders and ask loudly 'are you all right?'

  If they respond, keep them still, find out what's wrong and get help if needed.

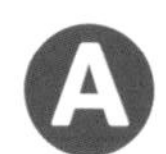

Airway

- Turn the casualty onto their back if necessary and open the airway:
  - With your hand on the forehead and fingertips under the chin, gently tilt the head back, lifting the chin to open the airway *(see picture)*.

B Breathing

- Look, listen and feel for **normal breathing** for **no more** than 10 seconds.

A casualty who is barely breathing, or taking infrequent, slow and noisy gasps is **NOT** breathing normally.
If you are in any doubt, prepare to start CPR.

Sometimes a short episode of seizure-like activity occurs when the heart stops. Check breathing immediately as the seizure ends and start CPR if needed.

*If **you are certain** that the casualty **is breathing normally**, place them in the recovery position if needed (page 17) and complete the primary survey (pages 8–9).*

Continued on next page.

If breathing is absent or abnormal:

Call 999/112 and send for a defibrillator *(AED)*:

- Ask a helper to call or activate the speaker function on your phone so that you can **start CPR** while talking to the ambulance call handler.
- Send someone to find and bring back an **AED** if available. If you are on your own and the AED is not nearby, don't leave the casualty – start CPR.

C Circulation

Kneel at the side of the casualty and start chest compressions:

- Place the heel of one hand in the centre of the chest *(lower half of the breastbone)*, place your other hand on top and interlock fingers.
- Keep your arms straight and position yourself vertically above the casualty's chest.
- **Press down on the breastbone at least 5cm** but no more than 6cm.
- After each compression, release all the pressure on the chest, without losing contact between your hands and the breastbone *(chest compression)*.
- Repeat chest compressions at a rate of 100–120 per minute with as few interruptions as possible.

Place the heel of one hand in the centre of the chest, then the other hand on top.

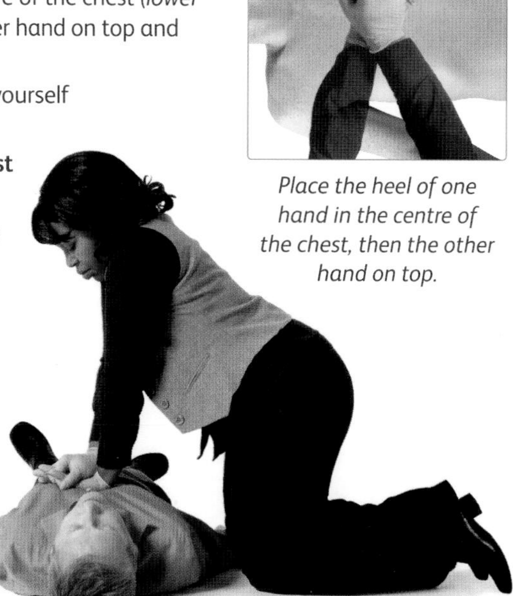

Arms straight and shoulders above your hands, depress the chest 5–6cm.

Now give rescue breaths – *over the page*

NOTE: *Ideally the casualty needs to be on a firm flat surface to perform chest compressions (not a bed). One way to remove someone from a low bed is to unhook the bed sheets and use them to slide the casualty carefully to the floor. Get help if you can and be very careful not to injure yourself or the casualty. If you think it's too risky to move the casualty, remove the pillows and kneel on the bed next to the casualty to give CPR (this helps to compress the mattress with your own weight). Increase your overall compression depth to compensate for the mattress compression.*

Combine chest compressions with rescue breaths:

If you are trained to do so, after 30 compressions, open the airway again and give 2 rescue breaths:

- Pinch the soft part of the nose closed. Allow the mouth to open, but maintain chin lift.
- Take a normal breath and seal your lips around the casualty's mouth.
- Blow steadily into the mouth, while watching for the chest to rise, taking about one second, as in normal breathing *(rescue breath)*.
- Keeping the airway open, take your mouth away from the casualty and watch for the chest to fall as air comes out.
- Take another normal breath and blow into the casualty's mouth once more to achieve a total of 2 rescue breaths. Do not interrupt compressions by more than 10 seconds to give 2 breaths.
- Return your hands without delay to the centre of the chest and give another 30 chest compressions.
- **Continue with chest compressions and rescue breaths at a ratio of 30:2.**

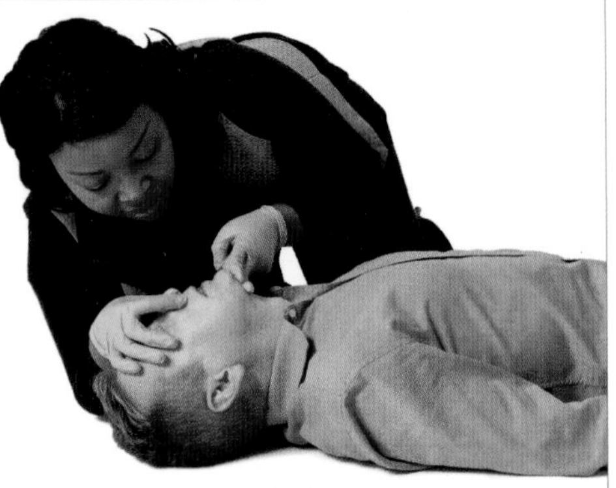

Pinch the nose.

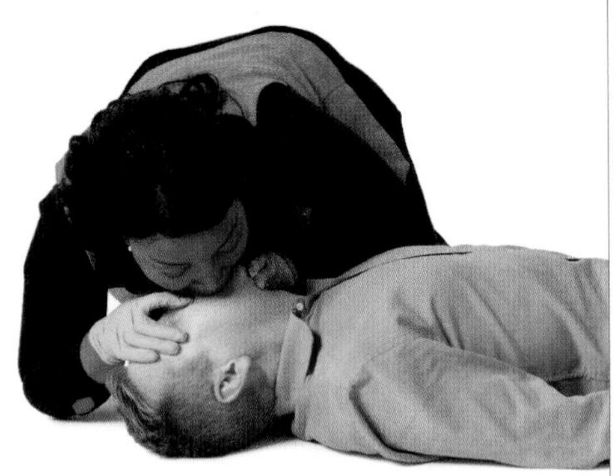

Rescue breaths.

If a defibrillator *(AED)* arrives – *continue to page 13*

More than one rescuer?

Change who does CPR every 2 minutes to prevent fatigue. Minimise delays when changing and **do not interrupt chest compressions**.

DO NOT interrupt CPR unless:

- A health professional tells you to stop;
- You become exhausted; **OR**
- The casualty is **definitely** waking up, moving, opening eyes and breathing normally.

When the defibrillator *(AED)* arrives:

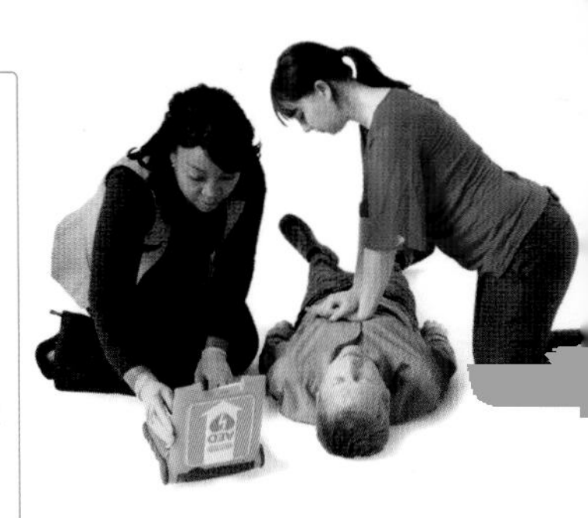

- If you have a helper, ask them to continue CPR whilst you get the AED ready. If they are untrained ask them to give chest compressions only *(page 14)*.

Switch on the AED immediately and follow the voice prompts:

- Attach the leads to the AED if necessary and attach the pads to the victim's bare chest *(do this whilst your helper performs CPR)*.
- You may need to towel dry or shave the chest so the pads stick properly. Only shave excessive hair and don't delay defibrillation if a razor is not immediately available.
- Peel the backing from one pad at a time and place firmly in position, following the instructions on the pads.
- Place one pad below the casualty's right collarbone.
- Place the other pad around the casualty's left side, over the lower ribs.

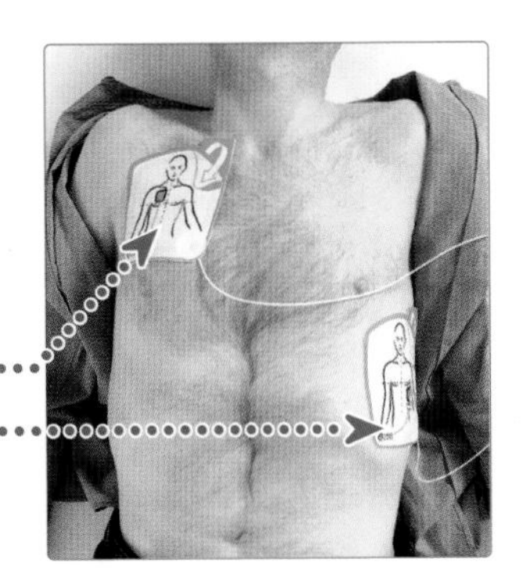

DO NOT *remove the pads if you have placed them the wrong way around – the AED will still work.*

- Whilst the AED analyses the rhythm – stop CPR and ensure that no one touches the casualty.

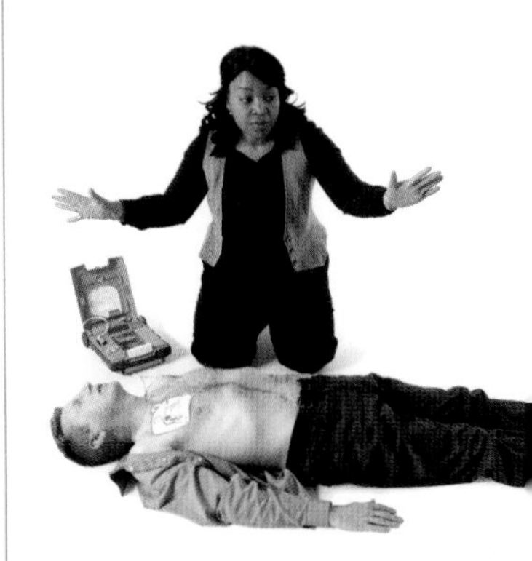

If a shock is advised, deliver shock:

- Make sure that nobody is touching the casualty.
- Push the shock button as directed *(fully automatic AEDs will deliver the shock automatically)*.
- Immediately restart CPR at a ratio of 30:2.
- Continue as directed by the voice/visual prompts.

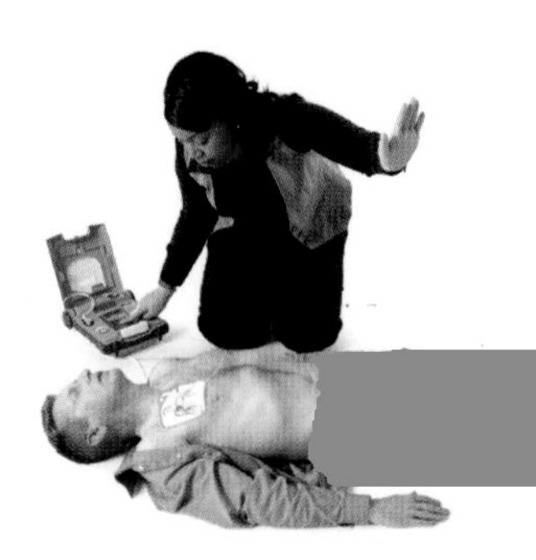

If a shock is NOT advised, continue CPR:

- Immediately restart CPR at a ratio of 30:2.
- Continue as directed by the voice/visual prompts.

Resuscitation for children and babies

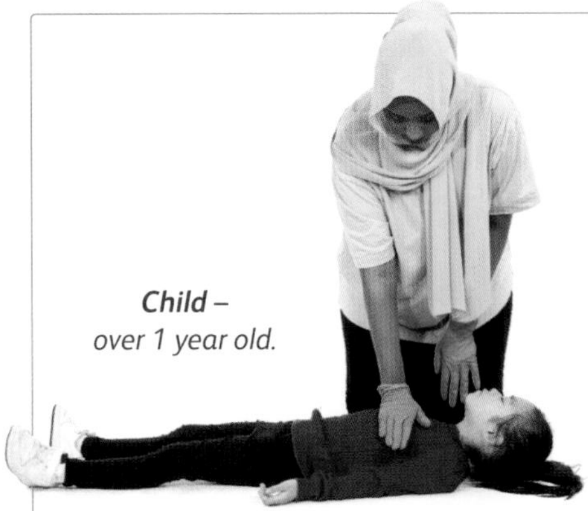

Child – *over 1 year old.*

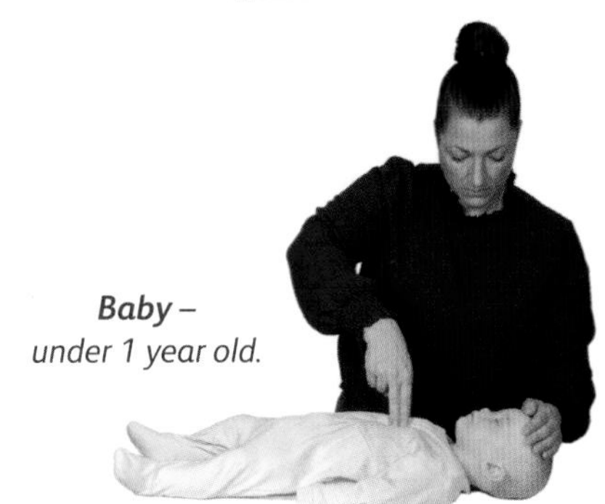

Baby – *under 1 year old.*

First aiders can use the **adult** sequence of resuscitation on a child or baby who is unresponsive and not breathing, compressing the chest to 1/3 of its depth. A child or baby is far more likely to be harmed if you do nothing.

The following minor modifications to the adult sequence, however, will make it even more suitable for babies and children:

- Give 5 initial rescue breaths before starting chest compressions.
- Compress the chest by at least one-third of its depth *(4cm for a baby and 5cm for a child)*:
  - **For a child** use 1 or 2 hands as required to achieve adequate depth. Change hands regularly *(or use both hands)* to prevent fatigue.
  - **For a baby** use 2 fingers.
- If you don't have a phone, give CPR for 1 minute before going for help.

Chest compression only CPR

If you are trained and able, it's best to give rescue breaths during CPR *(this is particularly important for children and victims of drowning)*.

If you are not trained, unable or unwilling to give rescue breaths, giving chest compressions only is far better than doing nothing, because it circulates any oxygen left in the blood.

- Give continuous compressions at a rate of 100–120 per minute.
- If there is more than 1 rescuer, change who does compressions every 2 minutes to prevent fatigue.

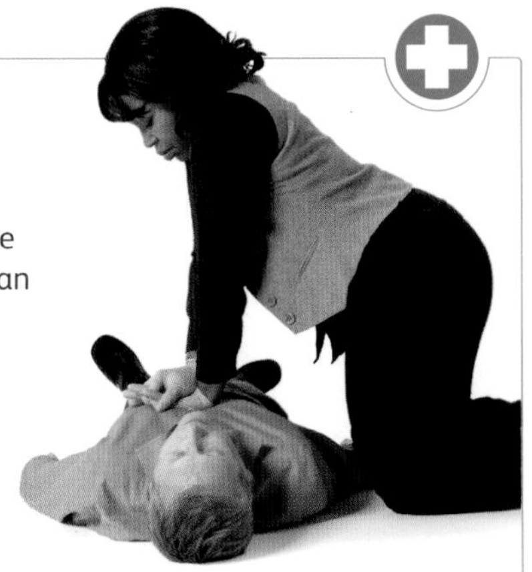

Vomit during resuscitation

Stomach contents are often regurgitated during CPR. This is a passive action, so you are unlikely to see or hear it happening. Vomit in the airway makes gurgling noises when you give rescue breaths. If this happens:

- Roll the casualty onto their side, tip the head back and allow the vomit to run out.
- Clean the casualty's face then continue CPR, using a protective barrier if possible.
- Minimise the interruption to CPR.

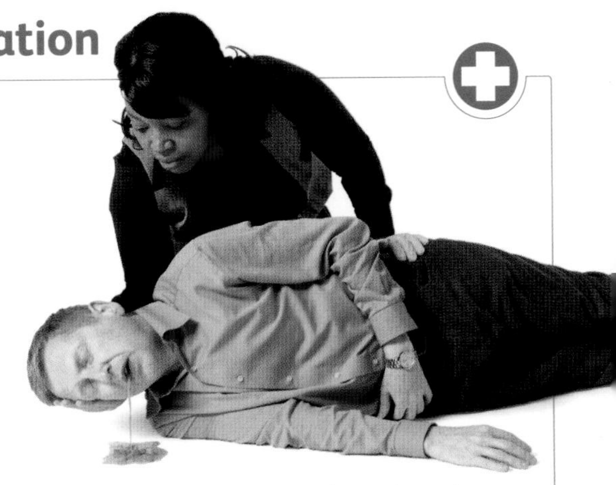

Turn them onto their side and allow the vomit to run out.

Hygiene during resuscitation

- For known or suspected COVID-19 infection, follow the COVID-19 CPR adaptations on page 64.
- If possible use a protective barrier such as a 'face shield' or 'pocket mask', however, this will not fully protect you from COVID-19.
- If you are still concerned about the safety of rescue breaths, give chest compressions only.
- Wear protective gloves if available and wash your hands afterwards.

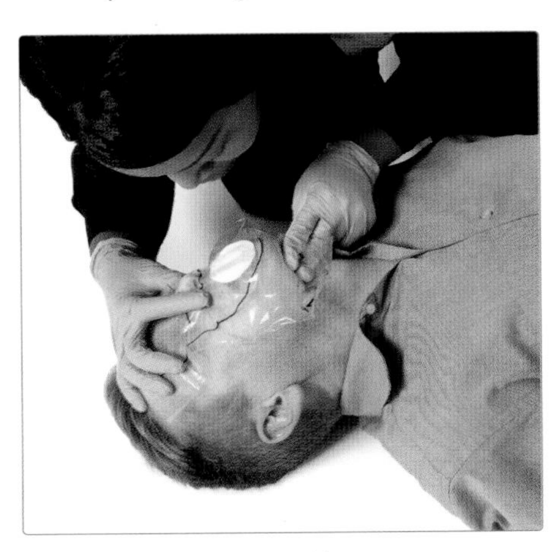

Face shield.

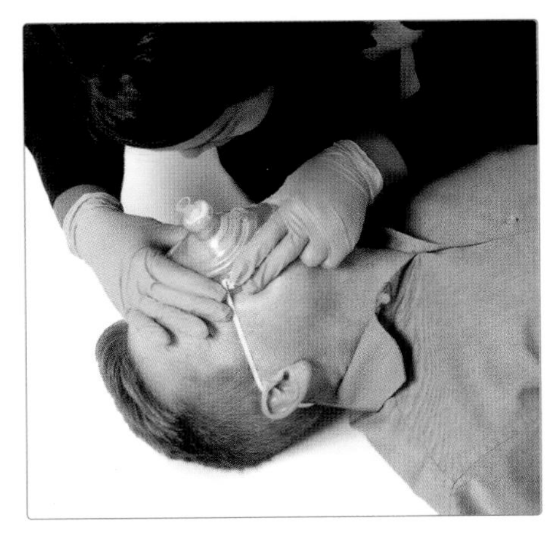

Pocket mask.

Unconscious casualty

Unconsciousness can be defined as 'an interruption in the normal activity of the brain'. Unlike sleep, unconsciousness can disable the body's natural reflexes such as coughing or gagging.

If someone is unconscious and laying on their back, the airway can become blocked by the:

- **Tongue** touching the back of the throat; **OR**
- **Vomit** if the casualty is sick.

For this reason, unconscious casualties take priority and need urgent help.

Placing a casualty in the **recovery position** *(opposite)* protects the airway from both of these dangers. The tongue will not fall backwards and vomit will run out of the mouth.

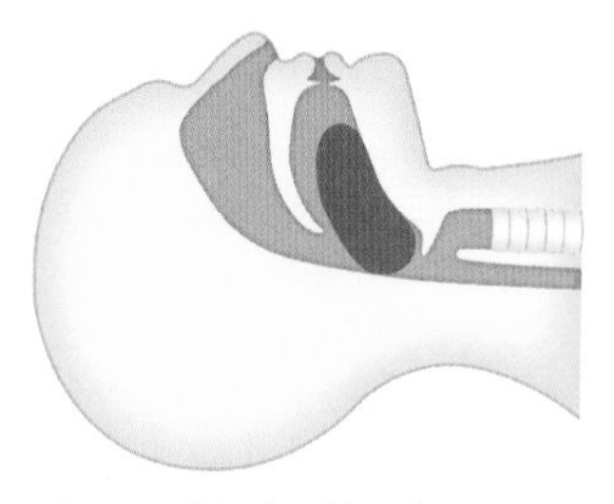

Airway blocked by the tongue.

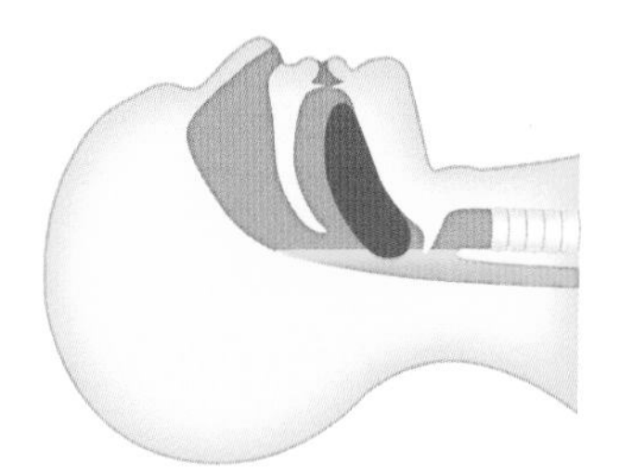

Airway blocked by vomit.

Levels of response

The simplest way to check if someone is conscious is to shout loudly, then gently shake or tap the shoulders. To measure the level of response, we can use the 'AVPU' scale:

A Alert	The casualty is fully alert. They can talk and will usually know what month it is.
V Voice	The casualty responds to your voice, but they are not fully alert.
P Pressure	The casualty responds to pressure stimuli or gently shaking the shoulders, but not your voice.
U Unresponsive	The casualty is unresponsive to pressure and speech stimuli.

Unconsciousness

Recovery position

The recovery position is intended for an unresponsive, uninjured casualty who is **breathing normally** *(does NOT need CPR)*. **For an injured casualty:** keep them still and continually monitor Airway and Breathing. Only use the recovery position if the airway is at risk *(e.g. fluids in the airway, or you have to leave them to get help and therefore cannot continually monitor breathing)*.

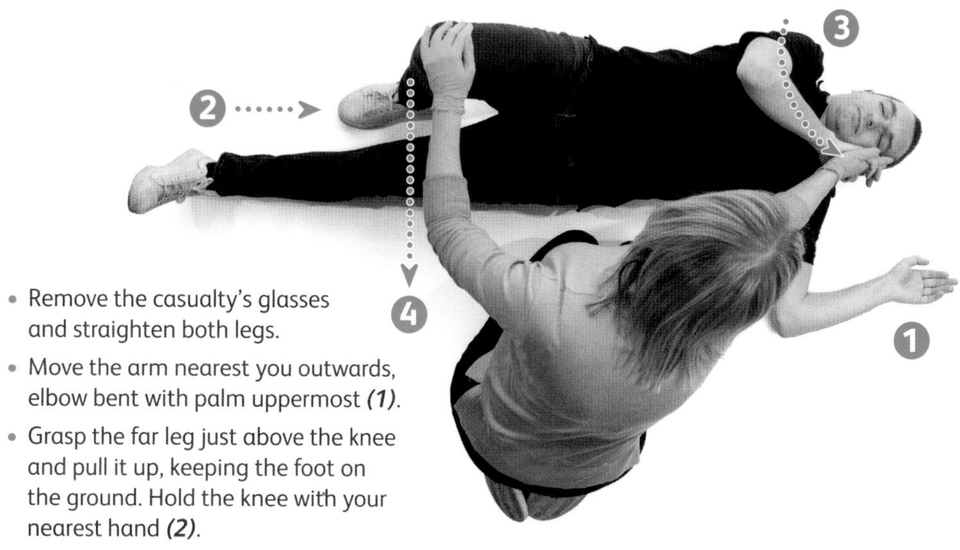

- Remove the casualty's glasses and straighten both legs.
- Move the arm nearest you outwards, elbow bent with palm uppermost ***(1)***.
- Grasp the far leg just above the knee and pull it up, keeping the foot on the ground. Hold the knee with your nearest hand ***(2)***.
- With your other hand, grasp the casualty's far hand palm to palm. Bring their hand across the chest and hold it against their cheek ***(3)***.
- Keeping the casualty's hand pressed against their cheek, pull on the leg to roll them towards you, onto their side ***(4)***.

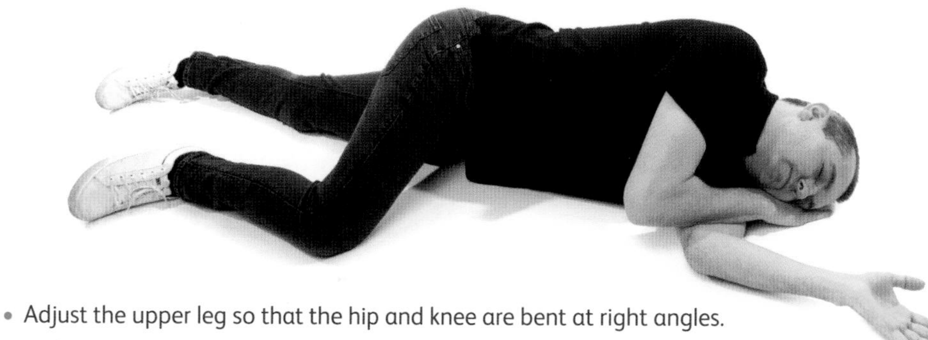

- Adjust the upper leg so that the hip and knee are bent at right angles.
- Make sure that the head is tilted and facing downwards to allow fluids to drain from the mouth.
- **Call 999/112 for emergency help.**
- **CONTINUALLY** monitor breathing until help arrives and start CPR if needed.

Seizures/epilepsy

Many things can cause a seizure – including epilepsy, reduced oxygen to the brain, stroke, head injury, or even a high temperature *(common in young children)*.

A major seizure often goes through a pattern:

Recognition

'Tonic' Phase

Muscles suddenly become rigid. The casualty may let out a cry and will fall to the floor. The back may arch and the lips can go blue. This phase typically lasts less than 30 seconds.

'Clonic' Phase

The arms and legs make sudden, rhythmical jerking movements, eyes may roll, teeth may clench, saliva can drool from the mouth *(sometimes blood-stained after biting the tongue)* and breathing could be noisy like snoring. There could be loss of bladder or bowel control. This phase typically lasts less than 2 minutes.

Recovery

The seizure stops but the casualty may still be unresponsive. They should wake within a few minutes but might not be 'alert' for 20 minutes or so.

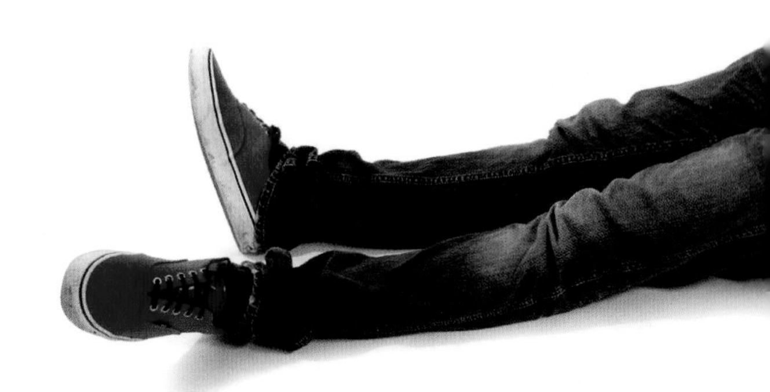

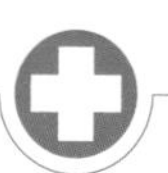

Treatment

During the seizure

- Move dangerous objects away and gently protect the head with a folded coat or your hands.
- Note the time and duration of the seizure.
- Loosen any tight clothing around the neck.
- **Call 999/112 for emergency help if:** the seizure lasts longer than 5 minutes, they have a second seizure, they have become injured or this is the casualty's first ever seizure.

After the seizure

- Open the **Airway** and check for normal **Breathing**. Start CPR if needed *(page 10)* or place them in the recovery position *(page 17)*.
- Move bystanders away to protect modesty.
- **Call 999/112 for emergency help** if you can't wake them up within 5 minutes.
- Constantly monitor **Airway** and **Breathing**.

NEVER place anything in the mouth.

NEVER try to restrain the casualty.

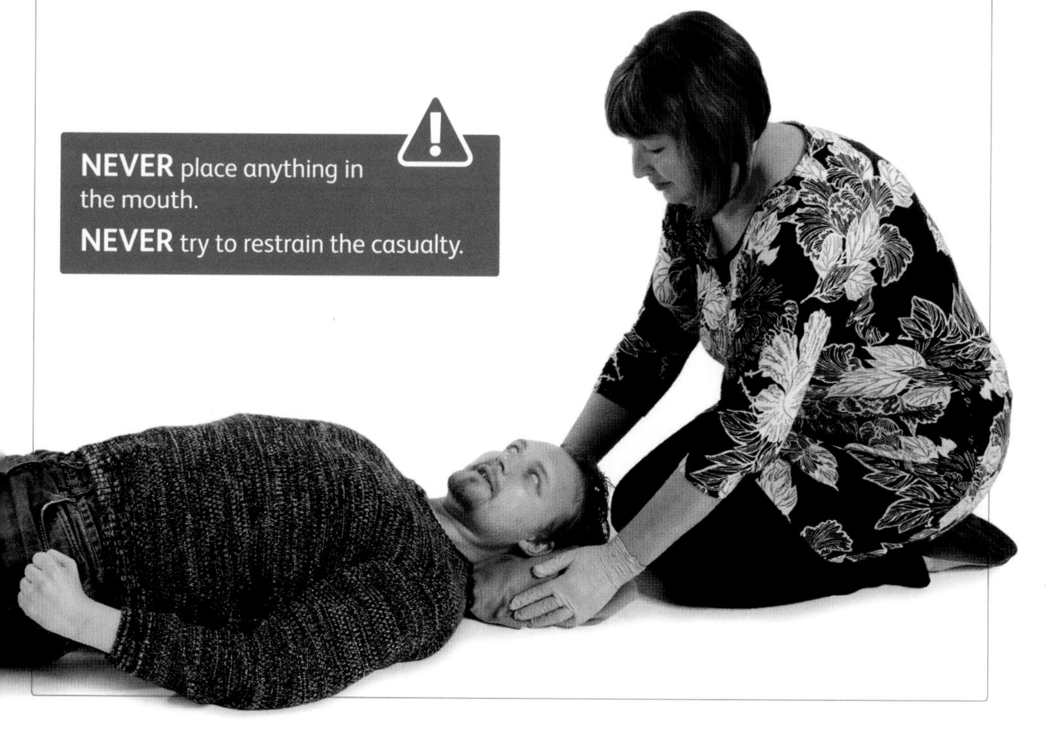

Choking

One of the most successful skills that a first aider can learn is the treatment of choking. Things such as food, sweets or small objects can easily become lodged in the airway if they are accidentally 'breathed in' rather than swallowed. Recognising that someone is choking is essential to a successful outcome.

Recognition

- Suspect choking if someone is suddenly unable to speak, particularly if eating.
- Ask the question: "Are you choking?"

Mild choking:

- If choking is mild, the casualty will be able to speak, cough and breathe.

Severe choking:

- Unable to cough effectively.
- Unable to speak – may 'nod' in response to your question.
- Struggling or unable to breathe.
- Distressed look on the face.
- Will become unconscious if untreated.

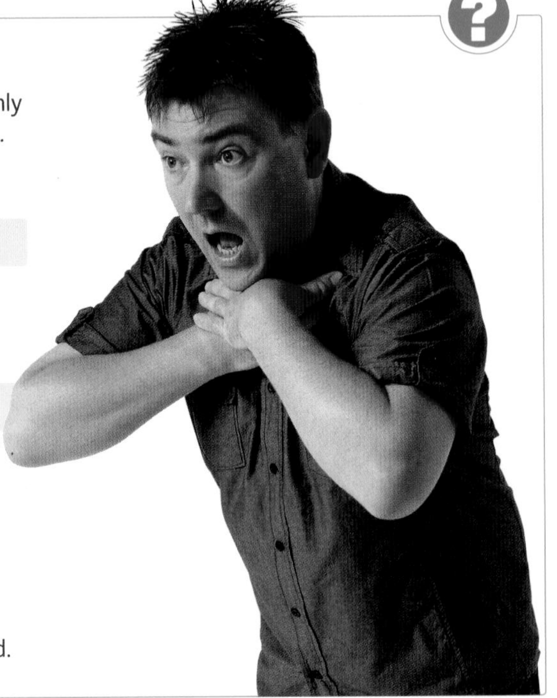

NEVER perform abdominal thrusts on a baby under 1 year old. Use chest thrusts instead.
See page 56 for Choking Baby treatment.

After successful treatment, seek immediate medical attention if the casualty: has received abdominal thrusts, chest thrusts or chest compressions; or has difficulty swallowing; or has a persistent cough; or feels like 'an object is still stuck in the throat'.

Treatment of choking – adult or child *(over 1 year)*

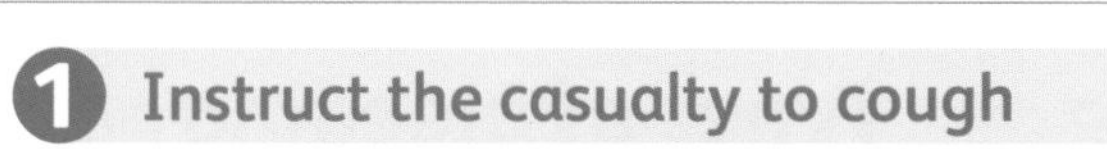

1 Instruct the casualty to cough

Instruct the casualty to cough. If the choking is only mild, this will clear the obstruction and they should be able to speak to you.

If the cough becomes ineffective:

2 Back blows

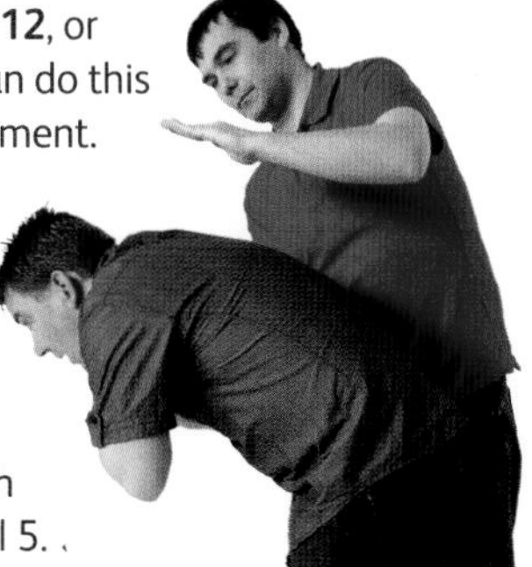

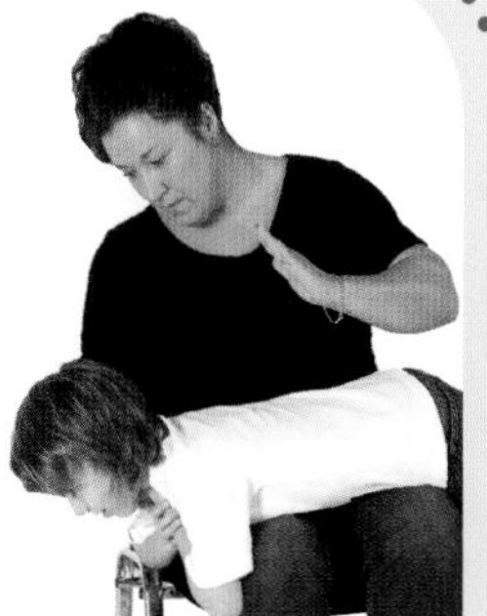

- Shout for someone to **call 999/112**, or call on a speaker-phone if you can do this at the **same time** as giving treatment.
- Lean the casualty forwards *(see pictures)*.
- Give up to 5 sharp blows between the shoulder blades with the heel of your hand. The aim is to relieve the choking with each blow rather than to give all 5. .

If the obstruction is still not cleared:

3 Abdominal thrusts

- Stand behind the casualty. Place both your arms around them.
- Make a fist with 1 hand and place it just above the belly button *(below the ribs)*.
- Grasp this fist with your other hand, then pull sharply inwards and upwards. Do this up to 5 times. The aim is to relieve the choking with each thrust rather than to give all 5.

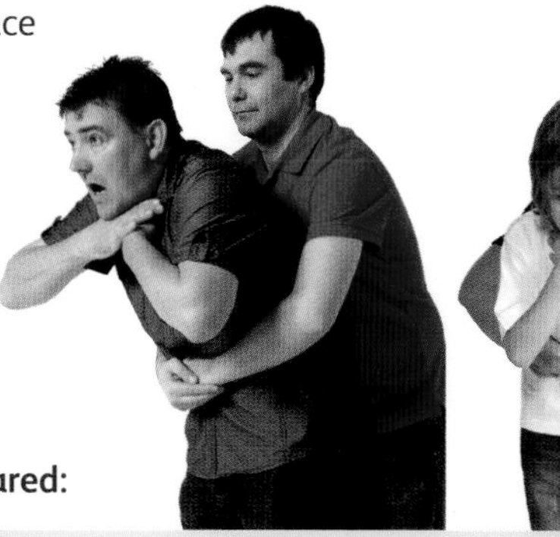

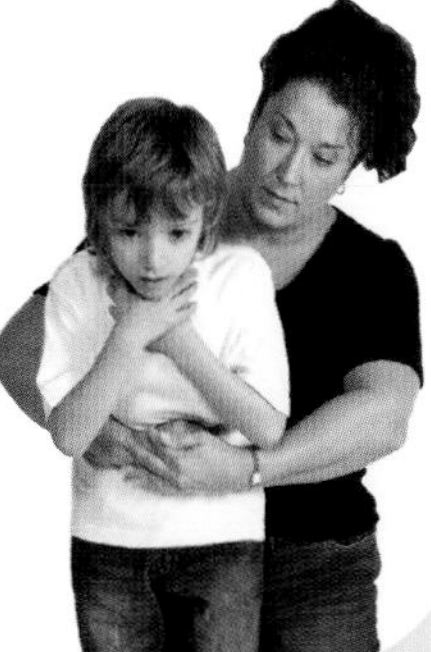

If the obstruction is still not cleared:

4 Repeat steps 2 and 3

- Keep repeating steps 2 and 3.
- If the treatment seems ineffective, make sure someone has **called 999/112 for emergency help**.

If the casualty becomes unconscious – START CPR *(pages 10–14)*.

Blood loss

How much blood do we have?

Our blood volume varies with our size, so a child has much less blood than an adult.

A rule of thumb is that we have around one pint of blood per stone in body weight *(0.5 litres per 7kg)* but the rule doesn't work if someone is overweight.

How much blood loss is critical?

The body compensates for blood loss by:

- Closing the supply to non-emergency areas *(e.g. the skin and digestive system)*.
- Speeding up the heart to maintain blood pressure.

There is a limit to how fast the heart can go and how many blood vessels can close, so the body cannot compensate after **one third** of the blood is lost. Beyond this, blood pressure falls quickly and the brain is starved of oxygen.

Remember – children have less blood than adults – just one third of a pint blood loss is life-threatening for a baby!

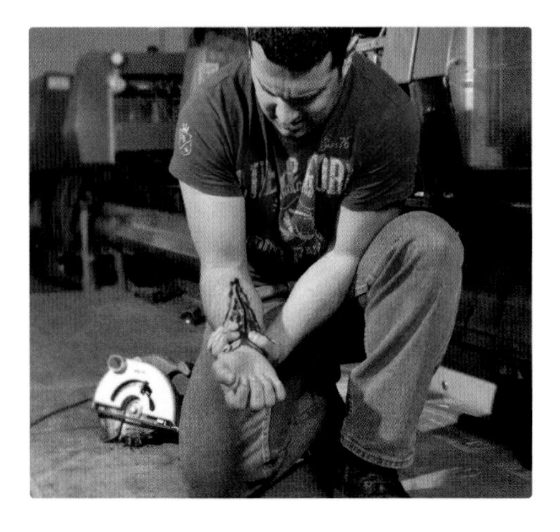

Types of bleeding

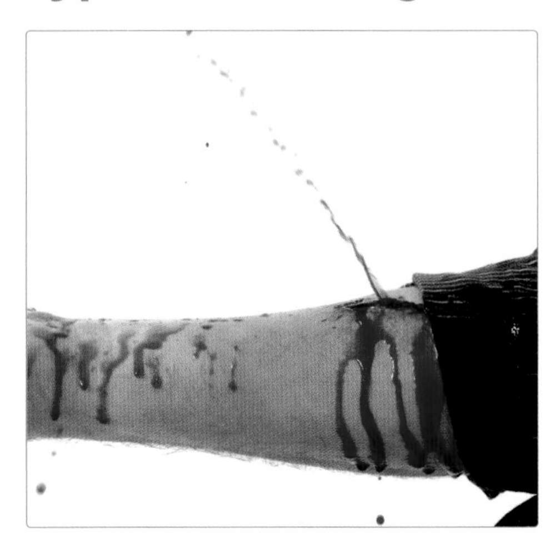

Arterial

Arterial blood is under direct pressure from the heart pumping and **'spurts'** in time with the heartbeat. Blood loss is rapid and can be life-threatening in just 2 minutes. Arterial blood is rich in oxygen and 'bright red', but this is difficult to assess. Looking at *how* the wound bleeds is easier.

Venous

Veins are not under direct pressure from the heart, but they carry the same volume of blood as the arteries. Bleeding from a major vein will **'flow'** profusely and is life-threatening.

Capillary

Bleeding from capillaries occurs in all wounds. Although the flow may appear fast at first, blood loss is usually slight and is easily controlled. Bleeding from a capillary could be described as a **'trickle'** of blood.

Shock

The definition of shock is *'a lack of oxygen to the tissues of the body, usually caused by a fall in blood volume or blood pressure'*.

Severe bleeding can result in shock, which can kill. If the casualty has lost a large quantity of blood this can cause a reduction in blood supply to the brain *(don't forget that children can't afford to lose as much blood as adults!)*.

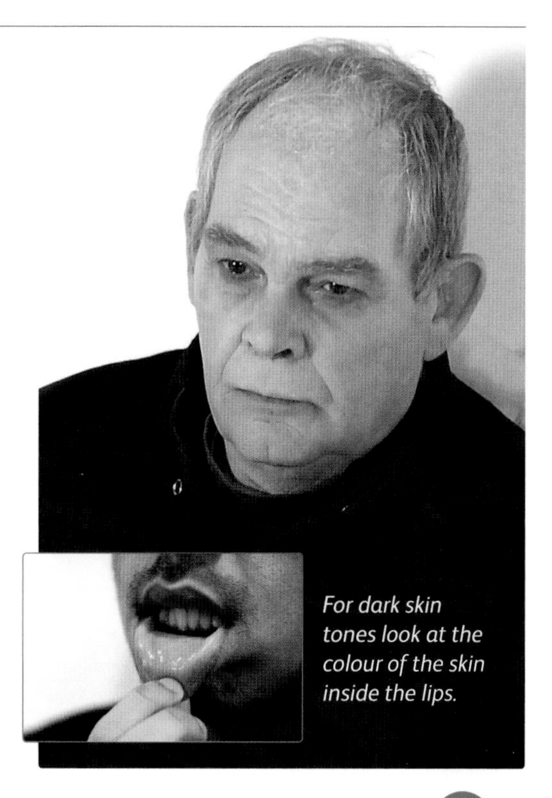

For dark skin tones look at the colour of the skin inside the lips.

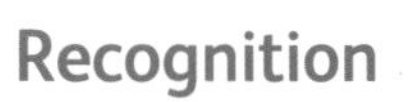

Recognition

- Pale clammy skin *(or pale skin inside the lips)* with blue or grey tinges if it's severe.
- Dizziness or passing out *(especially if they try to stand or sit up)*.
- A fast, weak pulse.
- Rapid shallow breathing.

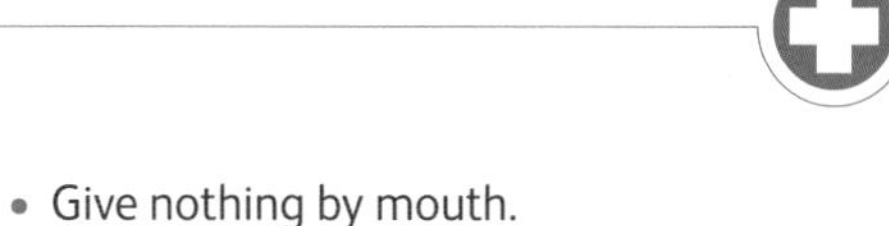

Treatment

- Treat the cause *(e.g. bleeding)*.
- Lay the casualty down. If there is no evidence to suggest broken bones, elevate the legs.
- **Call 999/112 for emergency help.**
- Keep the casualty warm *(but don't overheat them)*.
- Give nothing by mouth.
- Loosen tight clothing and monitor breathing.

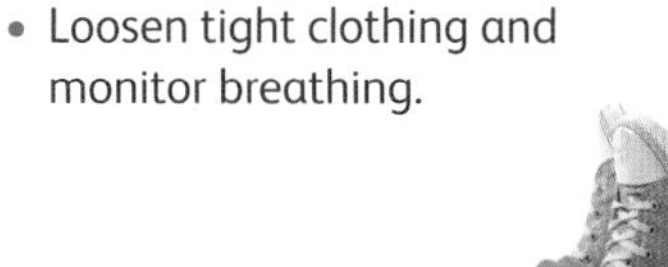

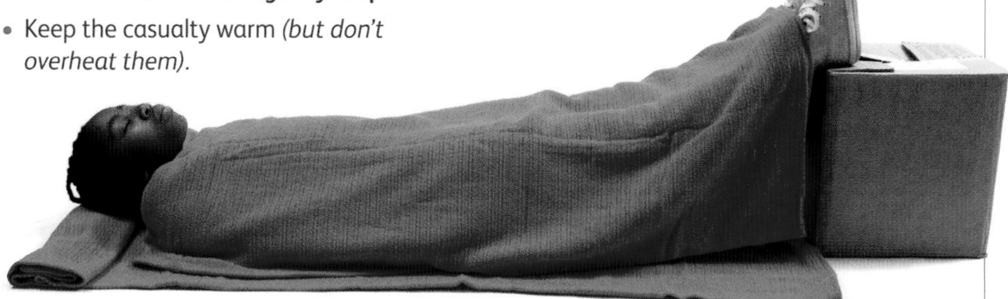

Treatment of bleeding

Sit or lay

Sit or lay the casualty down, appropriate to the location of the wound and the extent of the bleeding.

Examine

Very quickly note the type of bleeding *(arterial, venous or capillary)*. Identify the exact point of bleeding so you can apply pressure to the right spot. Look for foreign objects such as glass in the wound.

Pressure

Apply manual pressure to the point of bleeding **continuously for 10 minutes**. You may need to press **into** the wound. A deep wound may need packing to stop the bleed *(opposite page)*. If there is an embedded object, only apply pressure at either side and do not try to remove it.

Dress

You may be able to put a dressing on immediately and apply the direct pressure over it. A dressing should be sterile and just large enough to cover the wound. It should be absorbent and ideally have a surface that won't stick to the clotting blood *('low-adherent')*. The dressing should not restrict blood flow to the rest of the limb *(check the circulation at the far side of the dressing)*.

Pressure by hand will be necessary for severe bleeding. If a dressing gets saturated with blood, take it off and make sure you are applying direct pressure to the exact point of bleeding. Only re-dress it when the bleeding is controlled.

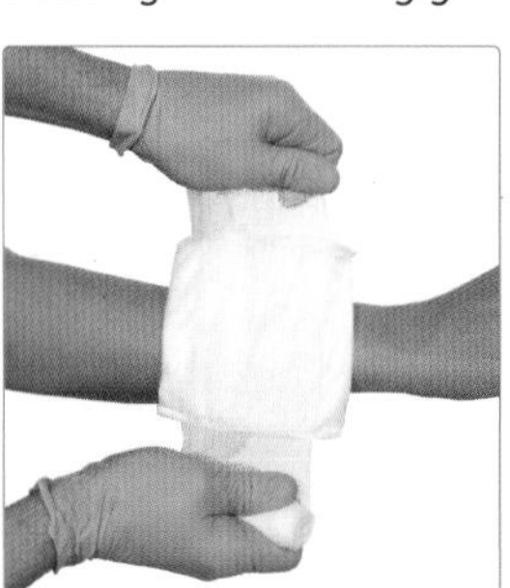

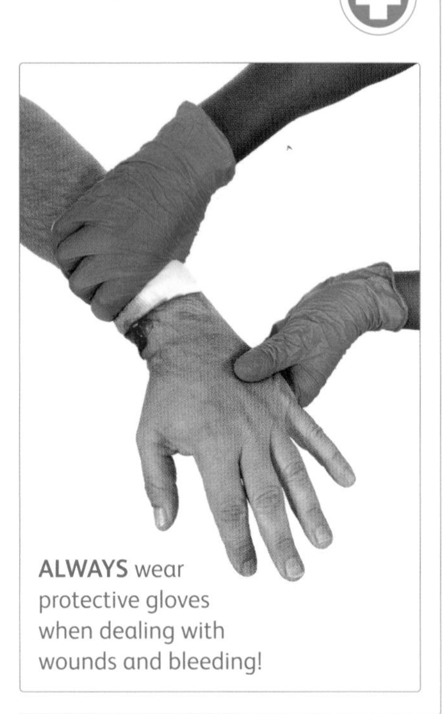

ALWAYS wear protective gloves when dealing with wounds and bleeding!

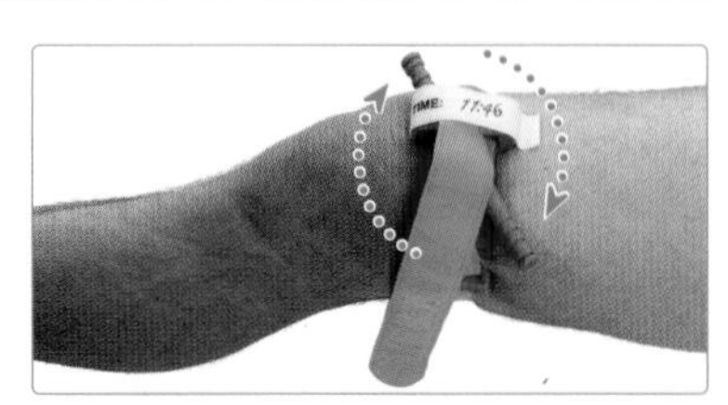

Manufactured tourniquet.

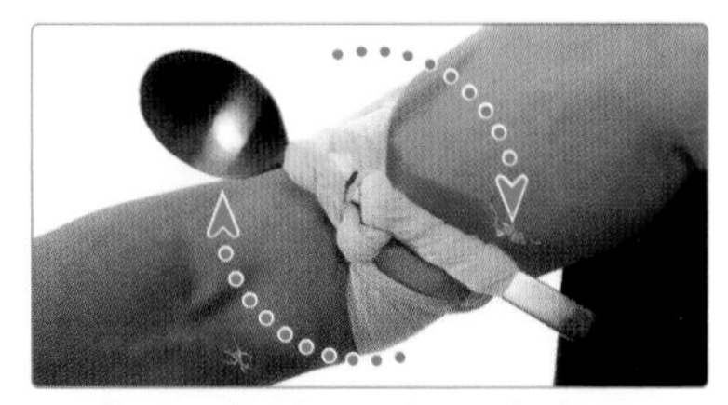

Improvised tourniquet (using a triangular bandage and a spoon).

Wound packing

If a wound is deep and bleeding heavily, it urgently needs packing tightly with a dressing or padding. For life-threatening bleeding, packing the wound with a 'haemostatic' dressing will control the bleeding faster as it contains an agent that rapidly and safely clots blood. **Any** packing however *(improvised if needed)* is far better than none!

Wound packing is often needed for life-threatening bleeding that cannot be controlled by direct pressure, such as deep wounds to the neck, groin or armpit. DO NOT pack a chest wound.

- Try to identify the exact point of severe bleeding and apply pressure. This may be **inside** the wound. Mopping out excess blood might help you find the exact place to press.
- Keeping pressure on the bleed, tightly pack the entire wound with the dressing and pack the *whole* dressing into the wound if you can.
- Manually press on the tightly packed wound for 10 minutes *(1 to 3 mins for a haemostatic dressing, see packet)*. Repeat if bleeding persists. Leave the packing in the wound and cover with another dressing. Send the haemostatic dressing packet to hospital with the casualty.

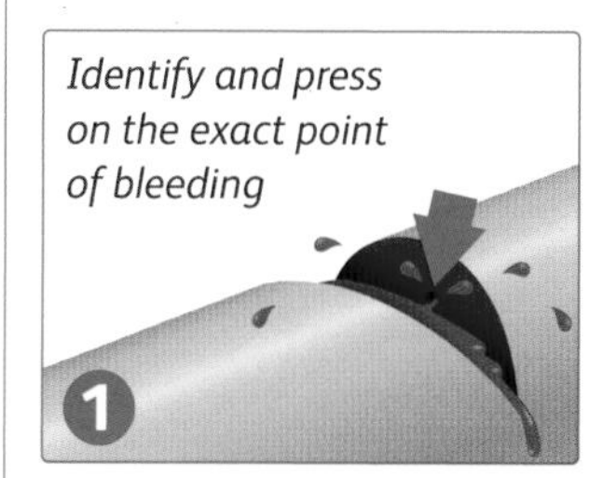

Identify and press on the exact point of bleeding

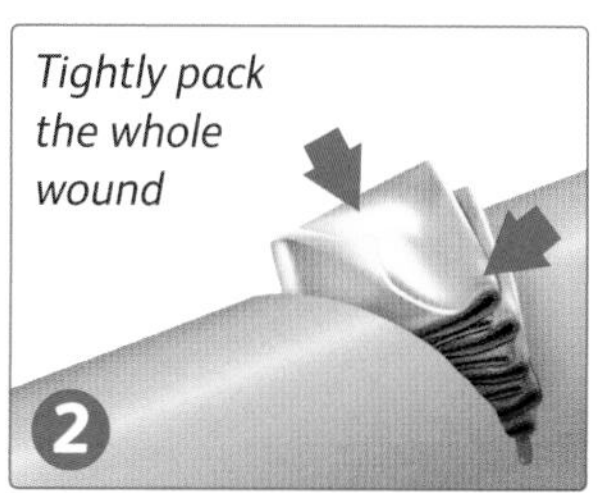

Tightly pack the whole wound

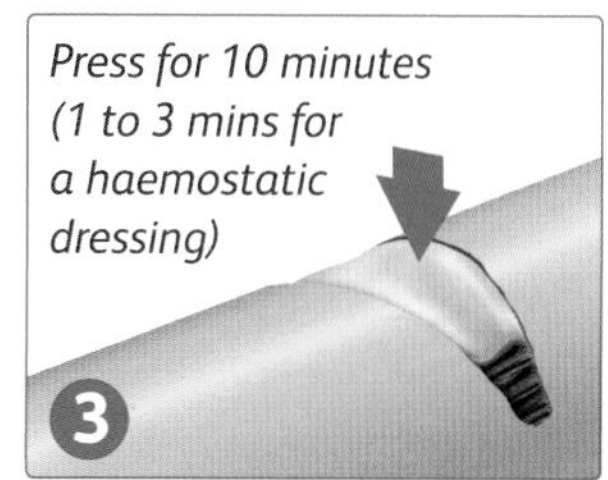

Press for 10 minutes (1 to 3 mins for a haemostatic dressing)

Tourniquets

A tourniquet is a band that is tightened around a limb to stop blood flow. Use a manufactured tourniquet for life-threatening bleeding from an arm or leg that cannot be controlled by applying manual pressure. If needed, it's okay to improvise using every-day items.

- Apply the tourniquet as rapidly as possible, directly to the skin, 5–7cm above the wound but not over the knee or elbow joint.
- Tighten the tourniquet until the life-threatening bleeding stops. This is painful for the casualty, so explain that this is needed to save their life.
- If the bleeding is not controlled: try tightening it more, reposition it, or apply a second tourniquet parallel to the first. Slight bleeding may still occur due to blood flow from the broken end of a bone.
- Make sure someone has **called 999/112 for emergency help**.
- Note the exact time of application and pass this information to medical staff.
- DO NOT release the tourniquet – this can only be done by a healthcare professional.

Warning: *if a tourniquet is not tightened enough it will squash the veins but not the arteries, which will actually make the bleeding worse!*

Minor injuries

Cuts and grazes

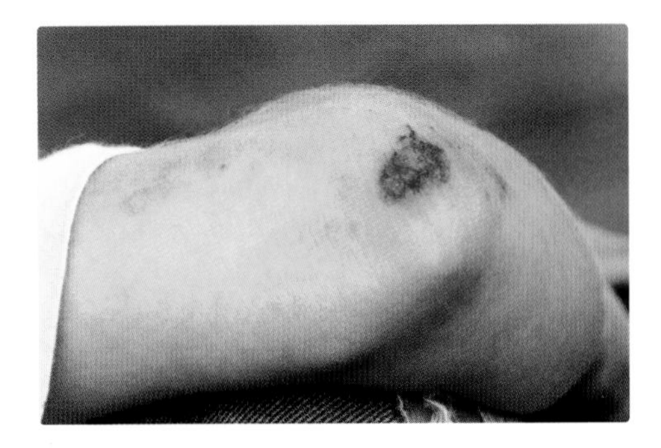

- Thoroughly irrigate superficial cuts and grazes with a large volume of drinkable water until there is no foreign matter in the wound. Slightly warm water can be more comfortable than cold. A little bleeding will help to wash out germs so don't worry.
- Pat the wound dry with a sterile swab then cover with a sterile plaster or low-adherent dressing.
- Seek medical advice if you are unsure if the casualty's tetanus immunisation is up to date.

Objects embedded in a wound

An object embedded in a wound *(other than a small splinter)* should not be removed as it may be stemming bleeding, or further damage may result.

Use sterile dressings and bandages to 'build up' around the object. This will apply pressure around the wound and support the object. Send the casualty to hospital to have the object removed.

Bruises

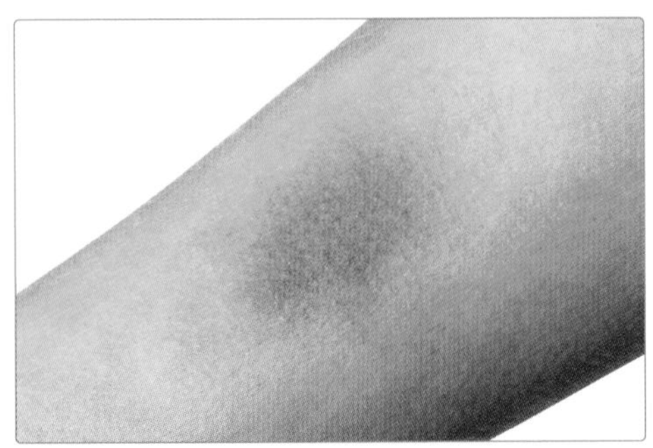

The main aim when treating a bruise is to reduce swelling.

- Wrap an ice pack in a tea towel or triangular bandage. Place it on the bruise and apply pressure for 10 minutes.
- If you don't have an ice pack, cold running water will help.

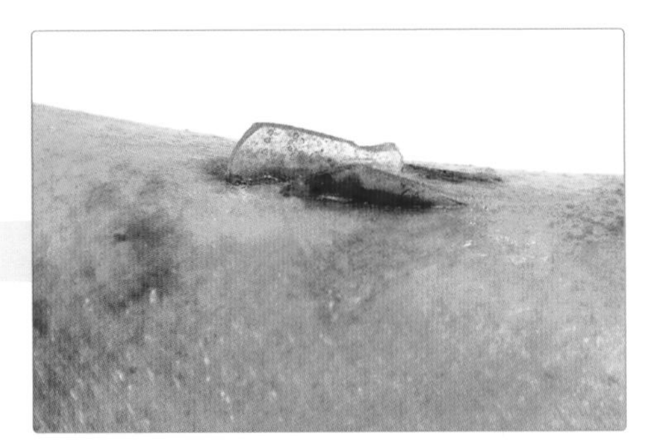

Objects stuck in the nose, ear or other orifice

Do not attempt to remove anything that someone has got stuck in their ear, nose or other orifice. Take them to hospital where the professionals can remove it safely.

Splinters

If a splinter is embedded deeply, difficult to remove or on a joint, leave it in place and follow the advice for embedded objects above. Other splinters can be removed as follows:

1 Carefully clean the area with warm soapy water.

Pat the area dry. Do not disturb the splinter.

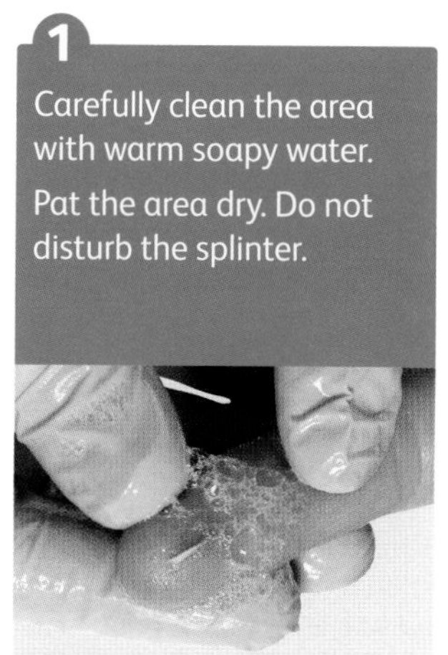

2 Using a pair of clean tweezers, grip the splinter as close to the skin as possible. Gently pull it out at the same angle that it entered.

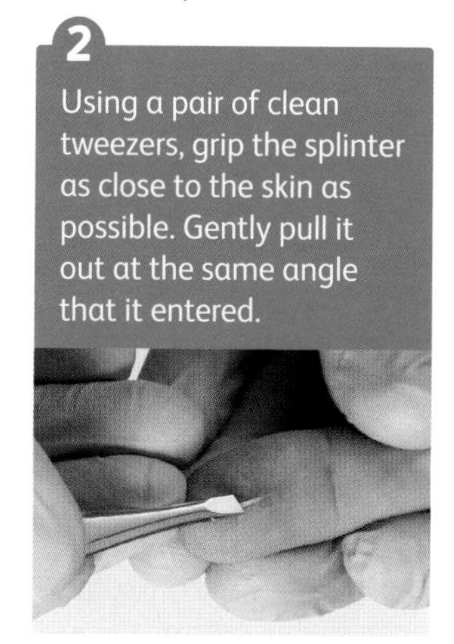

3 Gently squeeze around the wound to encourage a little bleeding. Wash the wound again, then dry and cover with a dressing.

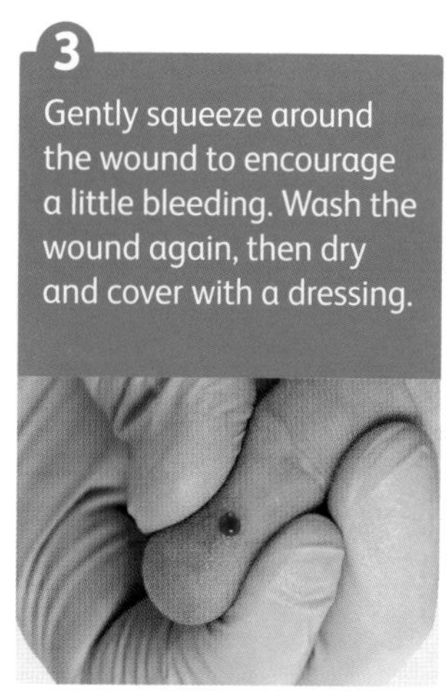

4 Seek medical advice to ensure the casualty's tetanus immunisation is up to date.

Insect sting *(bees and wasps)*

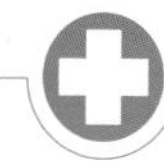

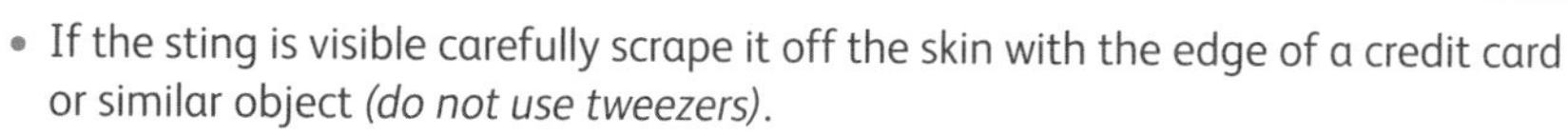

- If the sting is visible carefully scrape it off the skin with the edge of a credit card or similar object *(do not use tweezers)*.
- Elevate the injury if possible and apply an ice pack *(wrapped in a tea towel or triangular bandage)* for 10 minutes. Seek medical advice if the pain or swelling persists.
- If the sting is in the mouth, give an ice cube to suck on, or sips of cold water.
- Watch for allergic reaction.

Animal *(or human)* bite

Animal or human bites can be infected with bacteria or viruses, so it's important to flush out the wound thoroughly to reduce the risk of infection.

- Irrigate the wound thoroughly with large quantities of water.
- Treat for bleeding if necessary *(page 24)*.
- Pat the wound dry and cover with a sterile low-adherent dressing.
- Seek medical advice. Take or send the casualty to hospital if the wound is large or deep.

Nosebleed

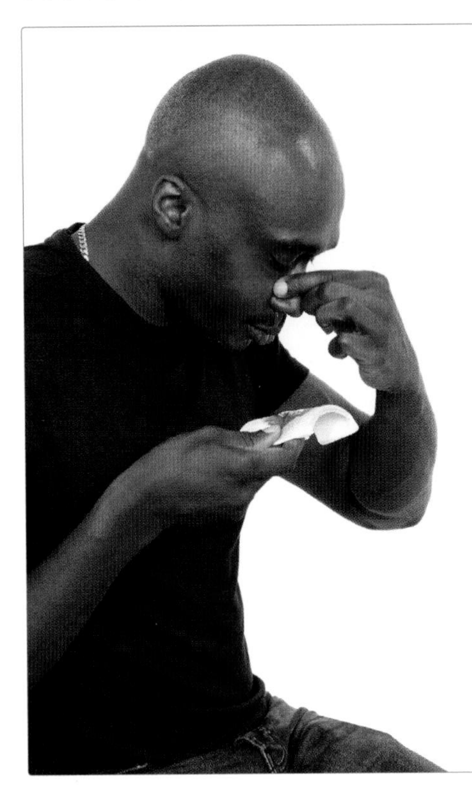

Weakened or dried out blood vessels in the nose can rupture as a result of a bang to the nose, picking or blowing it. More serious causes of a nosebleed could be high blood pressure or a fractured skull.

- Sit the casualty down, head tipped forward.
- Pinch the soft part of the nose. Maintain constant pressure for 10 minutes.
- Tell the casualty to breathe through the mouth.
- Give the casualty a disposable cloth to mop up any blood whilst the nose is pinched.
- Advise the casualty not to breathe through the nose for a few hours. Avoid blowing or picking the nose and hot drinks for 24 hours.
- If bleeding persists for more than 30 minutes, or if the casualty takes 'anti-coagulant' drugs *(such as warfarin)*, take or send them to hospital in an upright position.
- Advise a casualty suffering from frequent nosebleeds to visit their doctor.

Amputation

Amputation is the complete or partial severing of a limb, and is extremely traumatic for the casualty. Your priorities are to stop any bleeding, to carefully preserve the amputated body part and to reassure the casualty.

- Rapidly control any bleeding *(pages 24–25)*.
- **Call 999/112 for emergency help.**
- Dress the wound with a 'low-adherent', non-fluffy dressing.
- Place the amputated part in a plastic bag and then put the package on a bag of ice to preserve it. Do not allow the amputated part to come into direct contact with the ice or get wet.

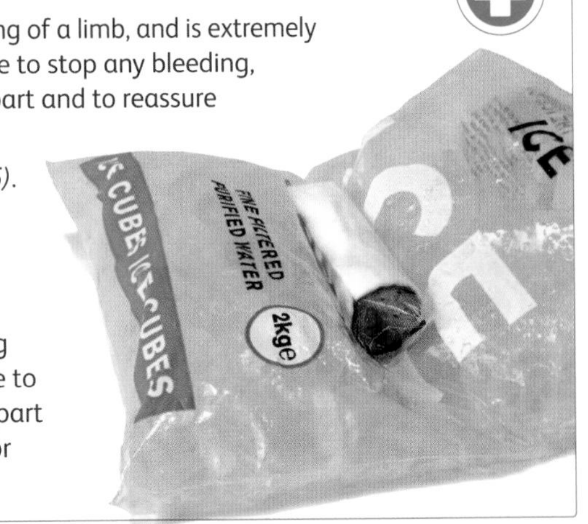

Penetrating injury

Causes of a penetrating injury can include being stabbed, shot or hit by shrapnel in an explosion. **Sometimes only a small entry wound is visible yet there can be deep internal damage.** Think carefully about which blood vessels and internal organs could be affected. With some injuries there can also be a large, crater-like exit wound.

- **Call 999/112 for emergency help** and make sure it is safe to approach.
- Control life-threatening bleeding as a priority:
  - Apply direct pressure to the exact point of severe bleeding if possible. This may be **inside** a deep wound. Tightly pack a deep wound with dressings *(use a haemostatic dressing if available, page 25)*.
  - For life-threatening bleeding to legs or arms – consider using a tourniquet *(page 25)*.
- Treat for shock *(page 23)*.

See also: Chest injuries, pages 38–39.

NEVER remove an embedded object – it might make the bleeding worse.

Minor burns and scalds

A minor burn is a common injury, such as a burn to the tip of a finger when cooking. The skin may be red and sore or there could be a blister.
For full information on burns see pages 44–45.

Cool the burn

Use cold running water for a full 20 minutes.

Immediate cooling is best, but is still beneficial even 3 hours after the burn.

Remove jewellery and loose clothing

Do this very gently, before the area starts to swell. Do not remove anything that is stuck to the burn.

Cover the burn

Cover the cooled burn with a dressing that won't stick. Cling film is ideal – discard the first two turns of the film and don't wrap it tight as the limb may continue to swell.

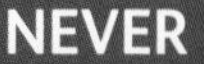

NEVER
- Apply ice
- Burst blisters
- Touch the burn
- Apply creams, ointments or fats
- Apply adhesive dressings
- Remove clothing that has stuck to the burn

Eye injuries

It is common for dust or dirt to blow in an eye and this is easily treated by a first aider. More serious injuries include chemical splashes, flash burns, embedded objects, tiny shards of glass or metal in the eye or larger physical damage.

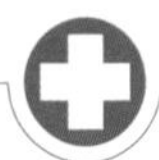

Treatment of eye injuries

Dust or dirt

- Small particles of dust or dirt can be washed out of an eye with cold tap water. Make sure the water runs away from the good eye.

For a more serious eye injury:

- Keep the casualty still and gently hold a soft sterile dressing over the injured eye. This can be carefully bandaged in place if necessary.
- Tell the casualty to close their good eye, because any movement of this will cause the injured eye to move too. If necessary bandage the good eye to stop the casualty using it. Lots of reassurance will be needed!
- Take the casualty to hospital. **Call 999/ 112 for emergency help** if necessary.

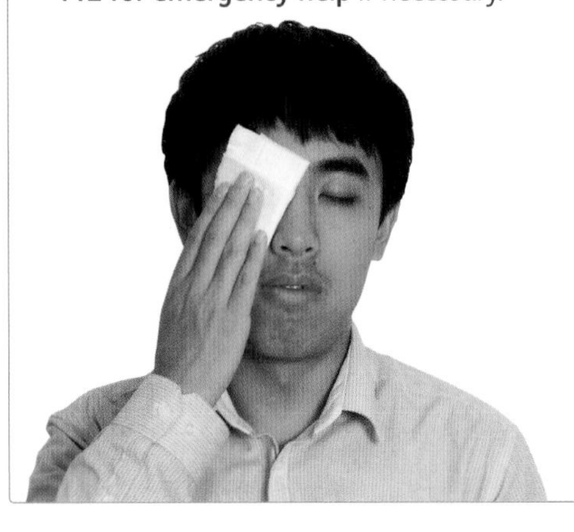

For chemicals in the eye:

- Irrigate with large volumes of clean water continuously, with the water running away from the good eye. Wearing gloves, gently, but firmly, try to open the eyelid to irrigate the eye fully. **Call 999/112 for emergency help**.

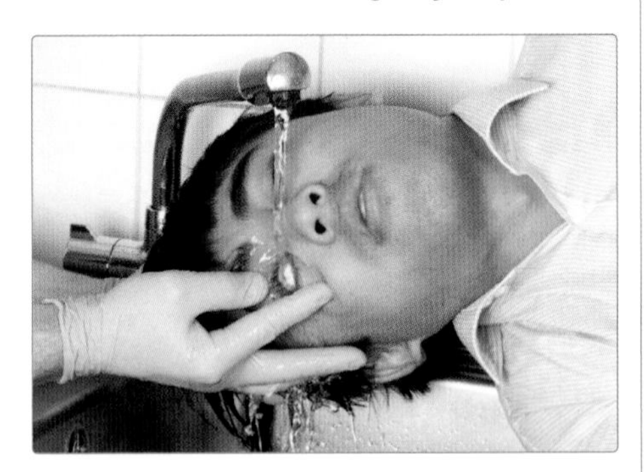

Flash burns to the eyes

Flash burns can occur from not protecting the eyes when looking at a welder's torch or prolonged exposure to the glare of the sun reflecting on the sea or snow. Intense pain in both eyes usually develops gradually, with sensitivity to light and a 'gritty' feeling in the eyes.

- Reassure the casualty and ask them to close both eyes. Cover with soft pads or a blindfold to keep out the light. Take or send the casualty to hospital.

The secondary survey

The primary and secondary surveys give a systematic way to prioritise urgent treatment and then thoroughly assess the casualty.

When the primary survey is complete *(pages 8–9)* and you have dealt with any life-threatening conditions, it is safe to examine the casualty head to toe, checking for other injuries or illness in a methodical manner.

If the casualty is unconscious, it is **VITAL** that you continually monitor and protect the **Airway**, **Breathing** and **Circulation** – these are the primary survey priorities to keep the casualty alive until emergency help arrives.

Start by considering the history, signs and symptoms:

History

What happened? What is the casualty's medical history? Is the casualty likely to have injuries?

Signs

Look for clues such as swelling, pale skin *(or pale skin inside the lips)*, deformity etc. Use all your senses.

Symptoms

If the casualty is conscious, ask how they feel. Do they have pain? Where is it? Can they describe it? Does anything make it worse or better? When did it start? How severe is it?

Does the casualty have any other feelings *(such as sickness, dizziness, feeling hot, cold or thirsty)*?

SAMPLE

'SAMPLE' can be used to remember some important things to ask the casualty:

S — **Signs and symptoms**
How do they look and feel?

A — **Allergies**
Do they have any?

M — **Medication**
Are they on any?

P — **Past medical history**
Do they have any?

L — **Last meal**
When and what?

E — **Event history**
What happened?

Head to toe check

Next check the casualty from head to toe. Protect their dignity and ask permission if possible. Wear disposable gloves and don't move them more than necessary.

The head to toe check is over the page

Head to toe check

1 Head and neck

- Has the casualty had an accident that might have injured the spine? *(page 40)*.
- Assess the breathing – is it fast or slow, shallow or deep, difficult or normal?
- Assess the pulse – is it fast or slow, strong or weak, regular or irregular?
- Check the size of the pupils. Are they equal?
- Check the whole head and face. Clues to injury could be bruising, swelling, deformity, bleeding or discharge from the ear or nose.

3 Abdomen

- Check the abdomen for abnormality or response to pain.
- Look for incontinence or bleeding.
- **DO NOT squeeze or rock the pelvis.**

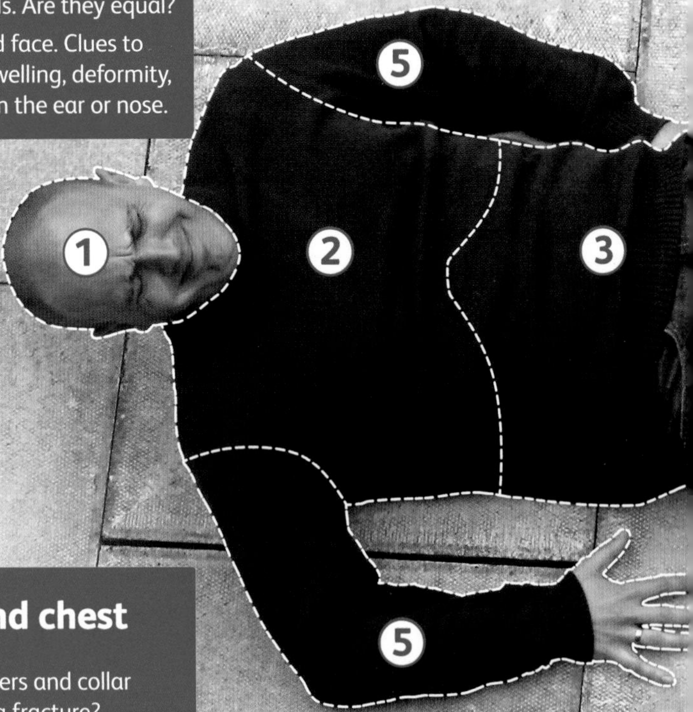

5

1

2

3

5

2 Shoulders and chest

- Compare opposite shoulders and collar bones. Are there signs of a fracture? *(page 34)*.
- Ask the casualty to take a deep breath:
  - Does the chest move easily and equally on both sides?
  - Does this cause pain?
- Look for injuries such as stab wounds or bleeding – front, side and back.

4 + 5 Legs and arms

- Ask the casualty if they can move their arms, legs and all the joints without causing pain.
- Check each limb for the signs of a fracture, deformity or bleeding.

6 Clues

- Look for clues such as medic alert bracelets, needle marks, medication etc.
- Loosen tight clothing.
- Have a reliable witness if you check or remove items from pockets or bags. Avoid this if you suspect there could be sharp objects such as needles.

4

4

CAUTION:

- If the casualty is unconscious, it is **VITAL** that you continually monitor and protect the **Airway**, **Breathing** and **Circulation** until emergency help arrives.
- If you suspect spinal injury, follow the advice on pages 40–41.

Broken or dislocated bones

Recognition

Pain	The injury usually hurts. Beware: pain-killers, nerve damage or other injuries can mask pain.
Loss of power	For example not being able to lift with a broken arm.
Unnatural movement	Take care to prevent movement if you see this.
Swelling or bruising	Around the site of the injury.
Deformity	If a bone is bent in the wrong place, it's broken!
Irregularity	Lumps or depressions in the skin where the broken ends of bone overlap or the bone has dislocated.
Crepitus	The feeling or sound of bones grating as the broken ends rub on each other if the injury is moved.
Tenderness	At the site of the injury.

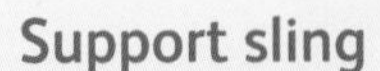

Support sling

A support sling is often used for supporting lower arm or collarbone injuries.

TIP: *Fold a triangular bandage in half for a small child.*

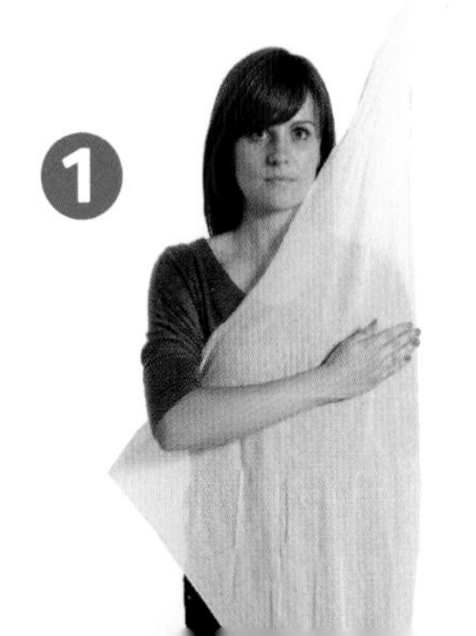

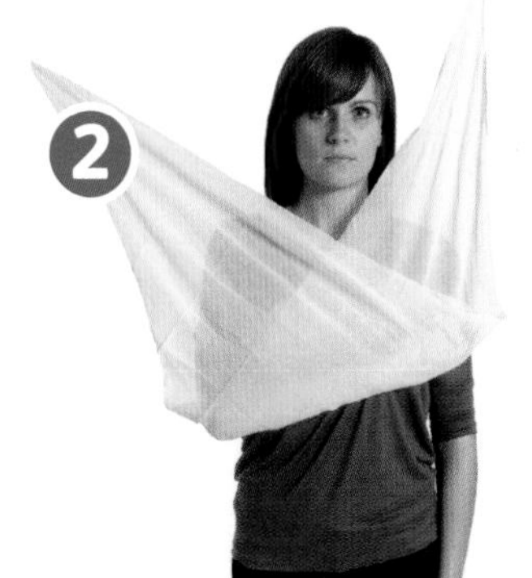

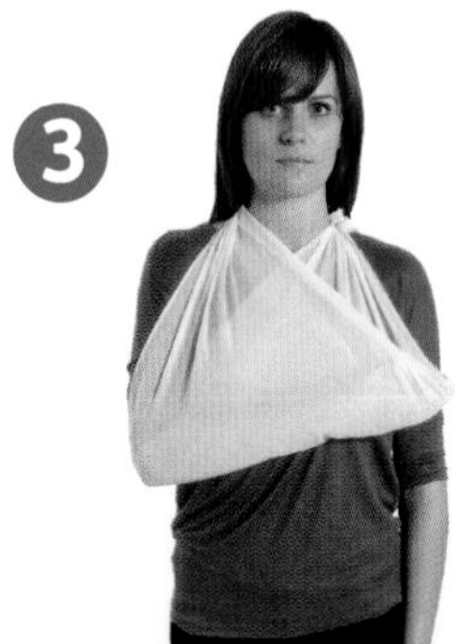

Treatment

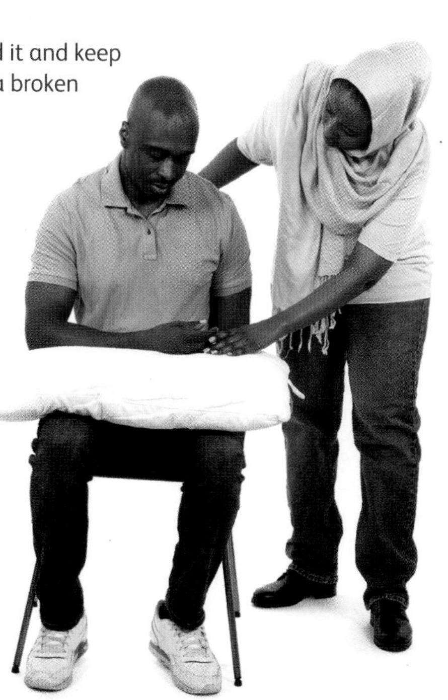

- Immobilise the injury in the position you find it and keep the casualty warm. Do not try to straighten a broken bone that is angulated.
- **Call 999/112 for emergency help if:**
  - You suspect injury to the spine or head.
  - There is difficulty breathing or reduced circulation beyond the injury.
  - There is deformity, irregularity, unnatural movement or bone through the skin.
  - The casualty is in a lot of pain.
  - You need help to safely immobilise the injury and transport the casualty.
- If you call 999/112, just keep the injury still and cover open wounds with a dressing.
- If you don't need an ambulance, splint/support the injury to immobilise it before transport to hospital. Pad inside any splint and check circulation beyond it.

Elevated sling

Elevated slings are often used for supporting rib injuries or for elevating a wound to the hand.

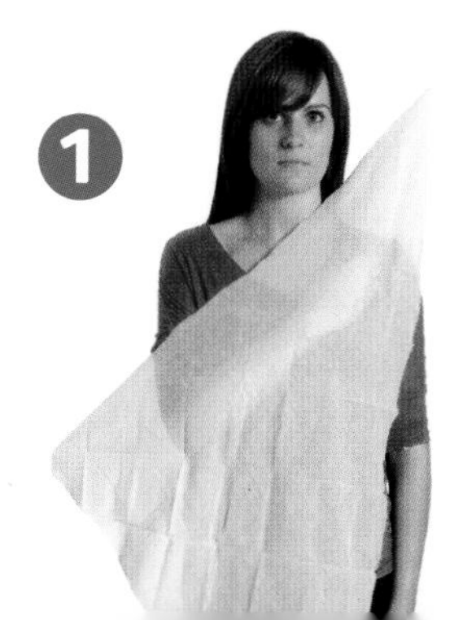

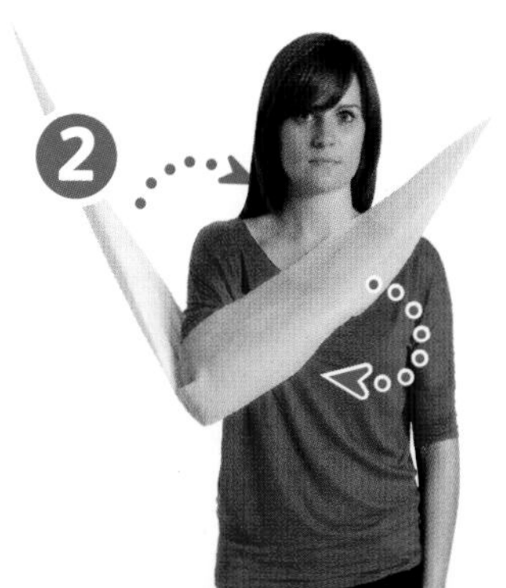

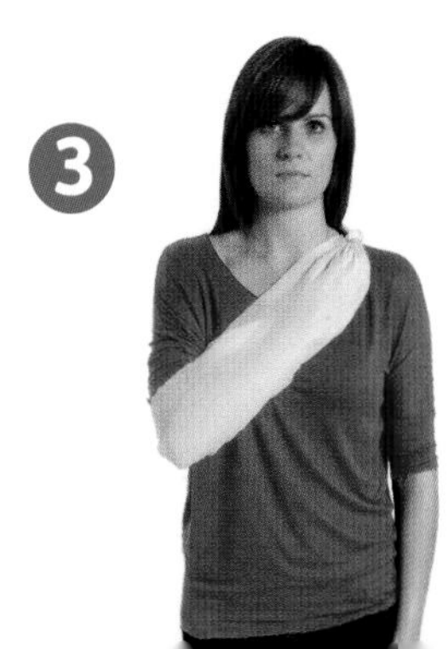

Sprains and strains

A **sprain** is an injury to a ligament at a joint and a **strain** is an injury to muscle. Usually caused by a sudden wrenching movement, the joint overstretches, tearing the surrounding muscle or ligament.

Recognition

- Pain
- Loss of power
- Swelling or bruising
- Tenderness

Minor fractures are commonly mistaken for sprains and strains. If you are not sure, treat the injury as a broken bone. Applying ice, however, will still help reduce swelling and pain. The only way to rule out a fracture is by X-ray.

Treatment

R **Rest** – Rest the injury and discontinue the activity that caused it. Protect it from further harm.

I **Ice** – Applying an ice pack can reduce pain and swelling. Place a damp tea towel or triangular bandage between the skin and the ice to prevent frostbite. Apply for a maximum of 20 minutes and allow the skin to return to normal temperature before repeating.

C **Compression** – Apply a firm *(not constrictive)* bandage to the injured area. This helps to reduce swelling.

E **Elevation** – Elevate the injury. This also reduces swelling.

REMEMBER: The only way to rule out a fracture is by X-ray, so take or send the casualty to hospital.

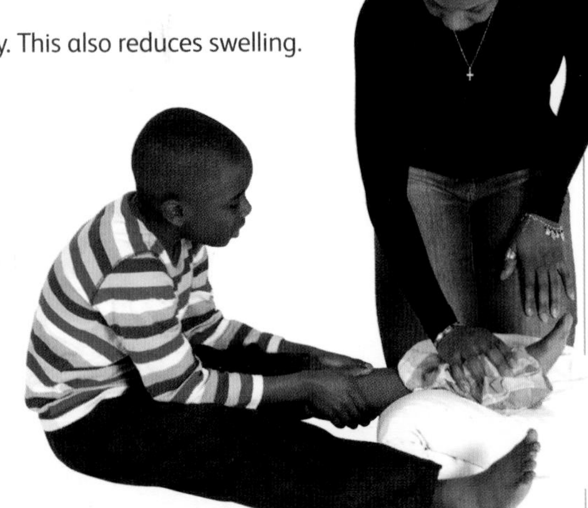

Chest injuries

Broken ribs

Ribs can break as a result of a fall or direct force. In serious cases, underlying organs such as the lungs, spleen or liver could be injured. Rib injuries that affect the breathing or cause internal bleeding can be life-threatening.

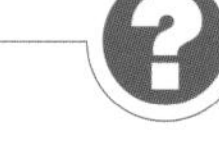

Recognition

- Pain
- Difficulty breathing
- Swelling or bruising
- Crepitus *(see page 34)*
- Tenderness

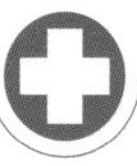

Treatment

- Place the arm on the injured side in a sling.
- Take or send the casualty to hospital.
- If the casualty has difficulty breathing or has signs of shock *(page 23)*, **call 999/112 for emergency help**.

Flail chest

This is a condition where the ribs surrounding the chest have become fractured in several places, creating a 'floating' section of the chest wall. As the casualty breathes, the rest of the chest wall moves out, but the flail segment moves inwards. As the chest wall moves back in, the flail segment moves outwards. These are called 'paradoxical' chest movements.

Recognition

- Severe difficulty breathing.
- Shallow, painful breathing.
- Signs and symptoms of a fracture *(page 34)*.
- 'Paradoxical' chest movements *(see above)*.

Treatment

- **Call 999/112 for emergency help.**
- Place the casualty in the position they find most comfortable – sat up, inclined towards the injury if possible.
- Place large amounts of padding over the flail area.
- Place the arm on the injured side in an elevated sling.

Collapsed lung

Both lungs and the inside wall of the chest cavity have separate linings, which together are called the 'pleura'. The lungs should fill the chest cavity, so the two linings should 'touch' each other, with just a thin layer of 'serous' fluid between them to help movement as we breathe. There should be no air or blood between the two linings.

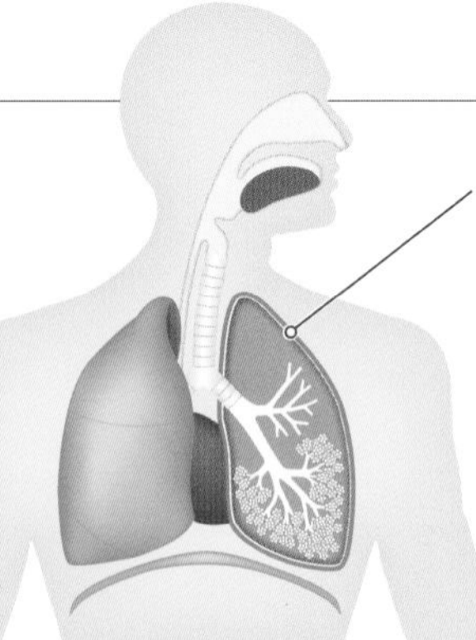

The pleural layers should be together with just a thin layer of fluid between.

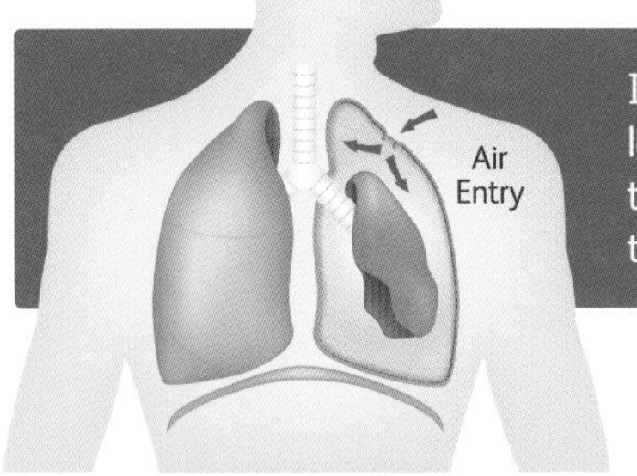

In a penetrating chest injury *(e.g. a stabbing)*, the outer layer of the pleura can be punctured and air can suck through the wound into the pleural cavity, causing the lung to collapse. The wound is called a **sucking chest wound**.

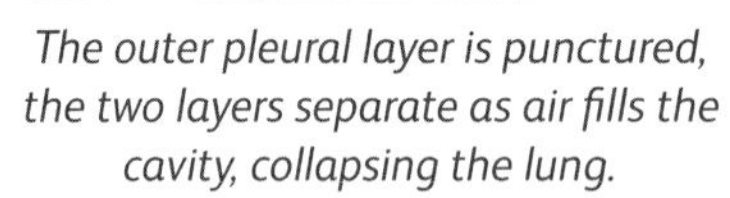

The outer pleural layer is punctured, the two layers separate as air fills the cavity, collapsing the lung.

Sometimes a penetrating injury can also perforate the inside layer of the pleura. Air can then escape from the **lung** into the pleural cavity, again causing it to collapse. Sometimes this inner layer can perforate when pressure is exerted on the lungs, such as the chest hitting the steering wheel in a car crash.

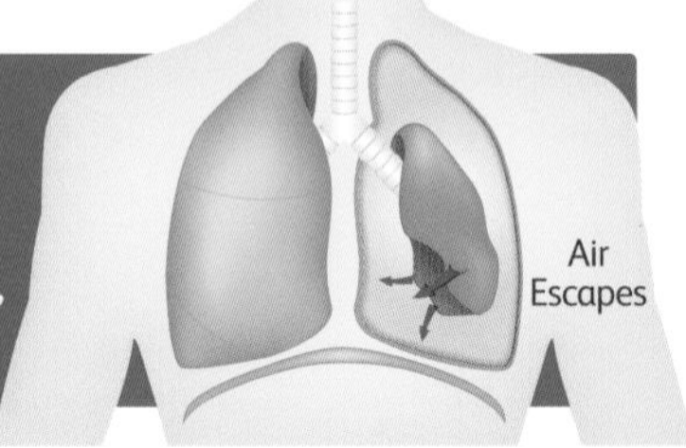

The inner pleural layer bursts allowing air to enter the cavity, collapsing the lung.

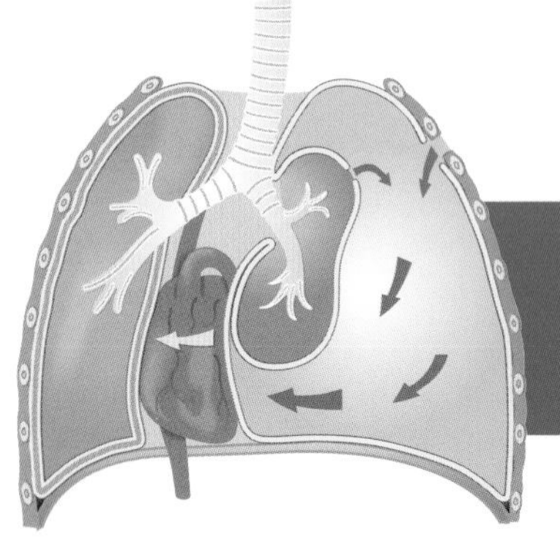

If air continues to enter the pleural cavity, **but does not escape**, pressure in the collapsed lung can build *(called 'tension pneumothorax')*. The pressure build-up can then squeeze the other lung and the heart, causing death.

Recognition

- Severe difficulty breathing.
- Painful breathing.
- Fast, shallow breathing.
- Blue tinges to lips and skin.
- Pale, clammy skin or for dark skin tones look for pale skin inside the lips.
- Uneven chest movements – the injured side of the chest may not rise.

If there is a sucking chest wound:

- Sound of air being drawn into the wound, with bubbling blood.
- Crackling sound if you press on the skin around the wound *(sounds like bubble wrap popping)*.

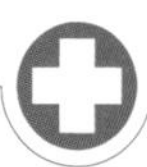

Treatment

- **Call 999/112 for emergency help.**
- If there are no other serious injuries, sit the casualty upright to help breathing, leaning towards the injured side.
- **If there is a sucking chest wound** – leave the wound open to fresh air if possible. It is important to allow air to escape to prevent tension pneumothorax. Apply direct pressure to stop bleeding but do not block the hole.

DO NOT *cover the hole with a dressing 'taped on 3 sides' as this can inadvertently occlude the hole. Specialised vented dressings are available but training is required in their use.*

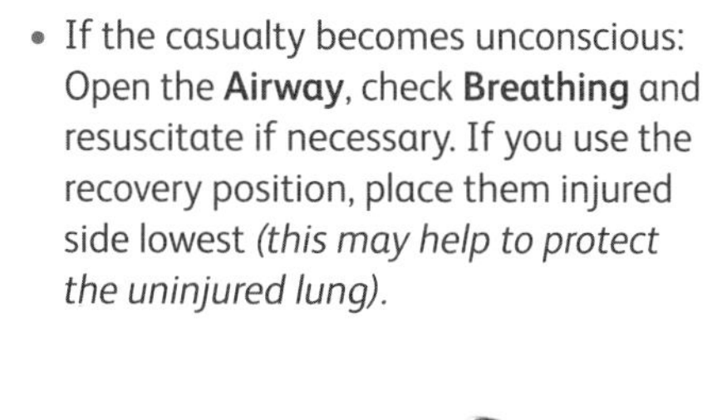

- If the casualty becomes unconscious: Open the **Airway**, check **Breathing** and resuscitate if necessary. If you use the recovery position, place them injured side lowest *(this may help to protect the uninjured lung)*.

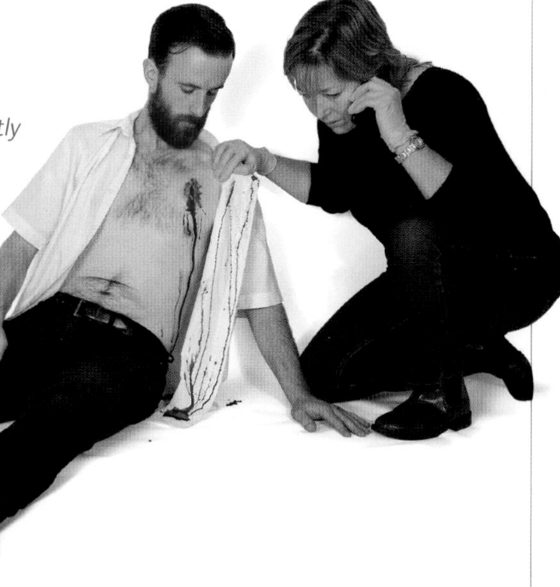

Spinal injury

The spine protects vital nerves that control movement and breathing, so if there is a possibility of spinal injury, correct treatment is vital. Look at the mechanics of the injury *(what happened to the casualty)* and if the incident suggests there could be a spinal injury, always treat for it.

Recognition

Suspect spinal injury if the casualty has:

- Sustained a blow to the head, neck or back *(especially resulting in unconsciousness)*.
- Fallen from a height *(e.g. from a horse)*.
- Dived into shallow water.
- Had an accident involving speed *(e.g. knocked down or a car accident)*.
- Had a 'cave in' accident *(e.g. crushing, or collapsed rugby scrum)*.
- Multiple injuries.
- Pain or tenderness in the neck or back after an accident *(pain killers or other injuries could mask the pain – beware)*.

If you are in any doubt, treat the casualty for spinal injury.

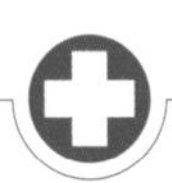

Treatment of suspected spinal injury

If the casualty is conscious:

- Offer reassurance and ask them not to move.
- Keep the casualty in the position you find them unless they are in danger. If necessary *(and they are able)* it's okay to allow a casualty to get themselves out of a vehicle.
- Tell the casualty to keep their head still, explaining that you are concerned about a broken neck. If needed, help them to do this.
- **Call 999/112 for emergency help**. Keep the casualty still and warm until help arrives.

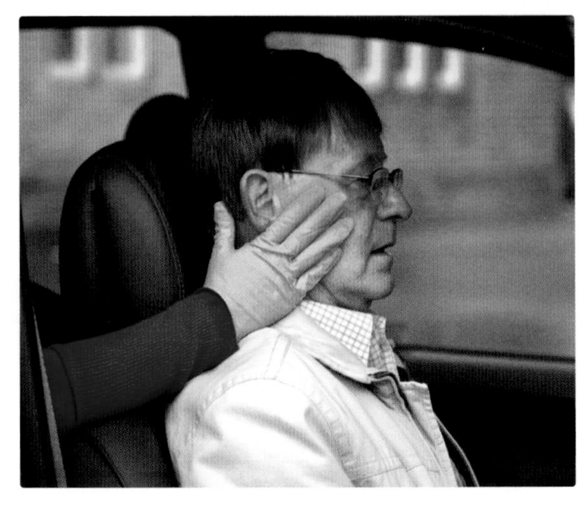

Helping a casualty to keep their head still in a car.

If the casualty is unconscious:

- If the casualty is **breathing normally** this means the airway must be clear, so there is no need to tip the head back immediately *(but you will have to tip it back and may need to resuscitate if they are not! See page 10)*.
- **Call 999/112 for emergency help.**
- Hold the head still. Keep the head and neck in line with the upper body.
- Keep the casualty warm and still. Continually monitor breathing until help arrives. Only move them if they are in danger.
- If there is an airway emergency *(e.g. the casualty is unresponsive, on their back and there are fluids in the airway)*, you may need to turn the casualty onto their side. **Keep the head and neck in line with the spine whilst you turn the casualty** *(see below)*.

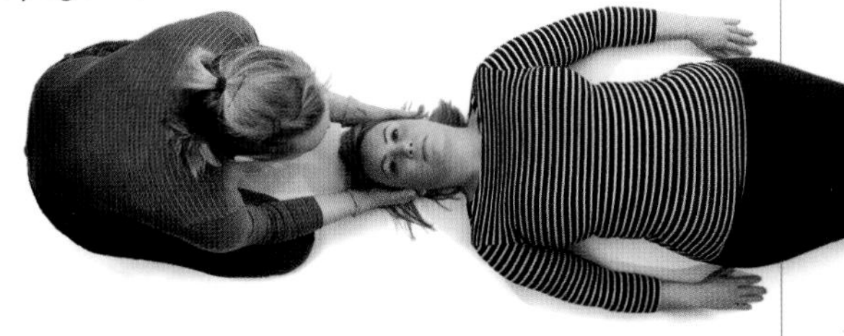

Spinal Recovery Position

Only move a spinal injury casualty if they are **unresponsive**, and the **airway is at risk** *(e.g. fluids in the airway)*.

If you need to turn the casualty due to an airway emergency, this spinal recovery position allows a lone-rescuer to quickly protect the airway whilst minimising movement of the spine.

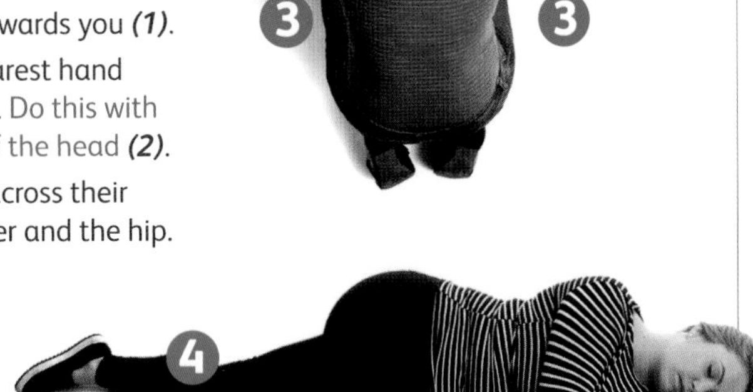

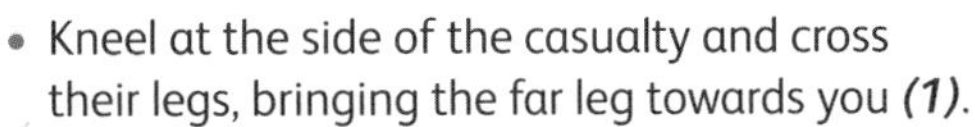

- Kneel at the side of the casualty and cross their legs, bringing the far leg towards you ***(1)***.

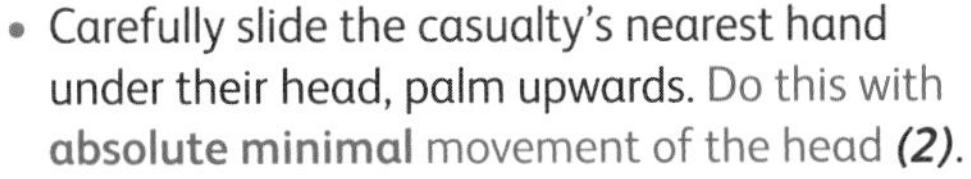

- Carefully slide the casualty's nearest hand under their head, palm upwards. Do this with **absolute minimal** movement of the head ***(2)***.
- Bring the far arm towards you, across their chest, then grasp the far shoulder and the hip.
- Pull **equally** on the shoulder and hip to roll the casualty towards you, onto their side ***(3)***.
- Adjust the upper leg so the hip and knee are at right angles ***(4)***.
- **CONTINUALLY MONITOR BREATHING** until emergency help arrives. Start CPR immediately if needed *(see page 10)*.

Serious head injuries

The three conditions concerned with serious head injuries are 'concussion', 'compression' and 'fractured skull':

Concussion

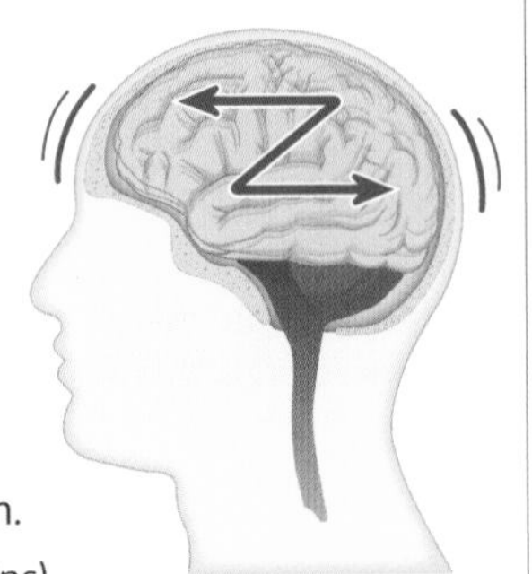

Concussion is caused by 'shaking' of the brain. The brain is cushioned within the skull by fluid, so if the head receives a blow the brain can bounce from one side to the other, causing widespread disruption to its normal functioning.

- The casualty may become **unconscious for a short period, after which the levels of response should improve**. The casualty should recover completely if no complications are present.
- Memory loss *(of the accident)* and repeating things is common.
- Other clues include pale, clammy skin *(or pale skin inside the lips)*, a mild general headache and nausea.

Compression

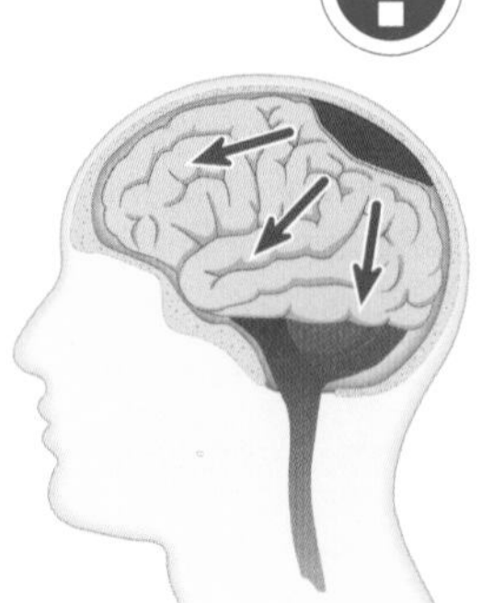

Caused by bleeding or swelling within the skull, compression is a very serious condition, because the brain is placed under extreme pressure *(see diagram)*.

- The casualty could have a history of recent head injury with apparent recovery, but then deteriorates. **Confusion and levels of consciousness become worse as the condition develops**.
- Other clues and symptoms include flushed, dry skin, intense headache and nausea.

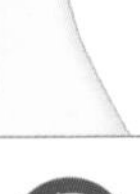

Fractured skull

A skull fracture is serious because the broken bone may directly damage the brain, or cause bleeding, which in turn results in compression. Suspect a skull fracture with any casualty who has received a head injury, especially if they have lowered levels of consciousness.

- **The casualty may also suffer from concussion or compression, so those signs and symptoms might be present.**
- Other clues include swelling or bruising of the head, around one or both eyes, or behind an ear.

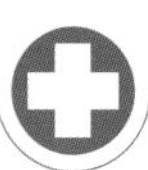

Treatment

REMEMBER: a blow to the head which is large enough to cause a head injury can also cause a spinal injury, so treat the casualty with care! *(pages 40–41)*.

- **Call 999/112 for emergency help** if the casualty has been unconscious, their levels of consciousness deteriorate, or you suspect a fractured skull.
- Maintain Airway and Breathing *(page 10)*.
- If the casualty is unconscious, keep them still and constantly monitor their breathing. If you are struggling to keep the airway clear, place them in the recovery position, but keep the head, neck and body in line as you turn them *(page 41)*.
- If the casualty is conscious, help them to lie down. Keep the head, neck and body in line in case there is a spinal injury.
- Control any bleeding by applying gentle pressure around the wound, but if there is bleeding or discharge from an ear, don't try to plug the ear or stop the bleeding.
- Look for and treat any other injuries.

Useful tips for head injuries:

- If you suspect concussion, arrange for the casualty to see a healthcare professional as soon as possible. Do not allow them to continue playing sports and stay with them until they are properly assessed.
- Constantly monitor and record breathing, pulse and the levels of consciousness.
- Even if the casualty appears to recover, watch out for a subsequent reduction in levels of consciousness *(as this could be the onset of compression)*. Although drowsiness can occur after a blow to the head, you should still be able to wake the casualty up.
- Seek medical advice before allowing the casualty to eat or drink.
- For the next few days, a casualty should go to hospital **immediately** if they suffer from: worsening headache, nausea, vomiting, increasing drowsiness, weakness in an arm or leg, speech problems, dizziness, bleeding or fluid from an ear or nose, visual problems, seizures or confusion.

Burns

Estimating the severity of a burn

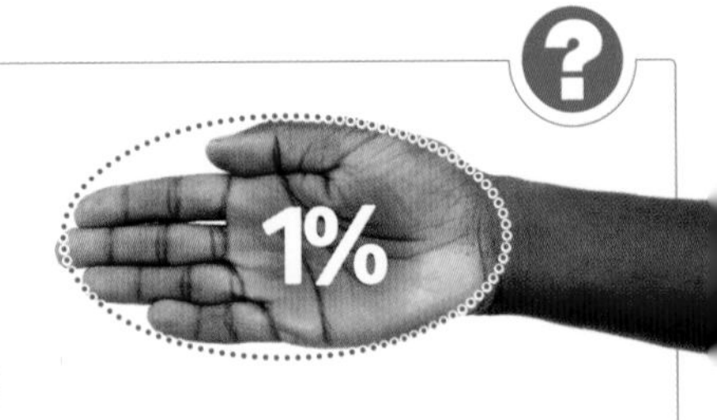

S Size — Any burn larger than 1% of the body area requires hospital assessment *(the same size as the palm of the casualty's hand including fingers)*.

C Cause — Causes include: Dry heat, wet heat *(scalds)*, radiation *(sunburn)*, chemicals and electricity. Chemicals could be poisonous and electricity can leave deep internal burns. Both require urgent hospital treatment. Chemicals should be washed off the skin for 20 minutes.

A Age — For children or the elderly, seek medical advice for any burn.

L Location — Burns to the face, hands, feet, genitals or burns that go all the way around a limb need hospital treatment.

D Depth — All full thickness burns should be treated in hospital *(see below)*. Always seek medical advice if you are unsure.

Depth of burns

The skin has 3 layers – the 'epidermis' on the outside, the 'dermis' beneath, then 'subcutaneous' fat. The depth of burns can be defined as:

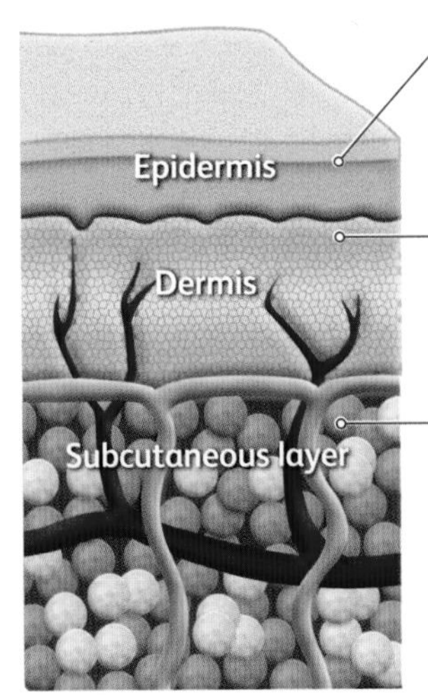

Superficial

Burns only the outer layer; often caused by hot water. It looks red, sore and swollen.

Partial Thickness

Burns both the epidermis and the dermis layers of skin. It looks raw and blisters form.

Full Thickness

The layers of skin are burned away to the subcutaneous fat layer or beyond. The burn may look pale, charred or waxy. The nerve endings will be burned away, so pain in this area may be absent, misleading both you and the casualty.

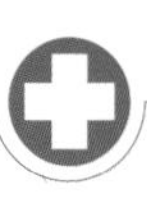

Treatment

1 Cool the burn

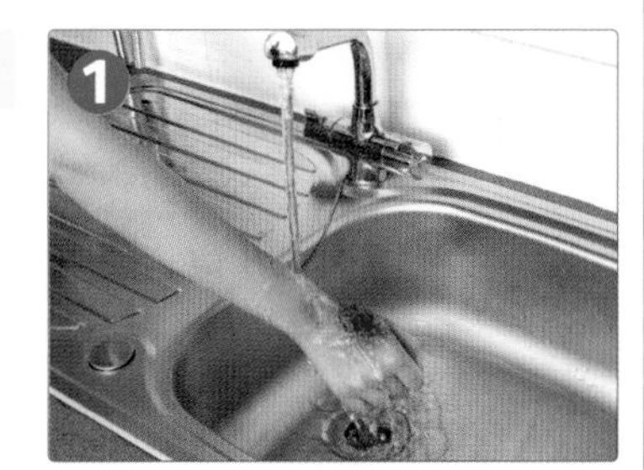

- Use cold running water for a full 20 minutes. Immediate cooling is best, but is still beneficial even 3 hours after the burn.
- Avoid hypothermia – cool the burn, but warm the rest of the casualty, especially the elderly or children.

2 Remove jewellery and loose clothing

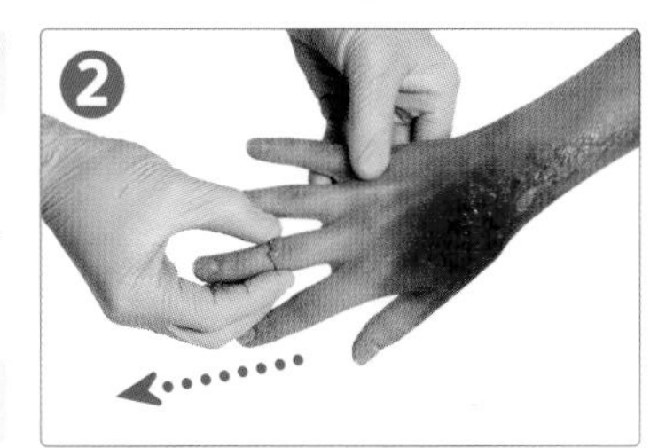

- Do this gently and carefully, before the area starts to swell. Do not remove anything that is stuck to the burn.

3 Cover the burn

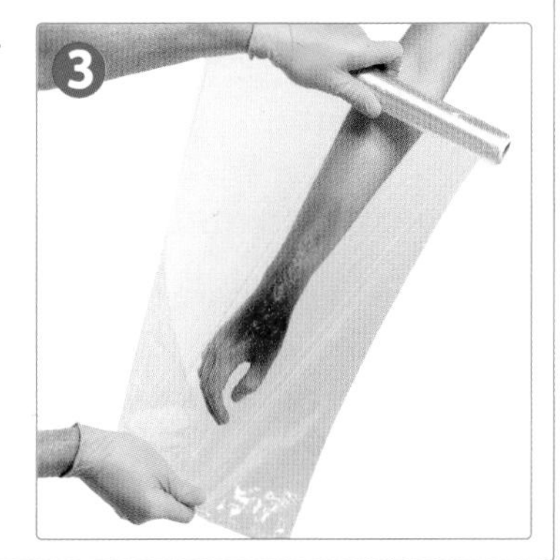

- Cover the cooled burn with a dressing that won't stick. Cling film is ideal *(discard the first two turns of the film and 'lay' it on the burn, don't wrap it around)*. Alternatives include a new *(unused)* plastic bag, a low-adherent dressing or a clean lint free cloth. Don't use cling film on the face.

  ***NEVER** rely on 'burn dressings' to cool a burn – use cold water for 20 minutes.*
- If the burn appears severe or the casualty has breathed in smoke or fumes, **call 999/112 for emergency help**.

NEVER:

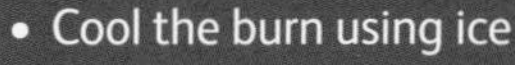

- Cool the burn using ice
- Burst blisters
- Touch the burn
- Apply creams, ointments or fats
- Apply adhesive dressings
- Remove clothing that has stuck to the burn

Chemical burns

Avoid contaminating yourself. Remove contaminated clothing, brush off dry powder/solid chemicals, then irrigate with running water for at least 20 mins. Avoid washing the chemical onto unaffected areas. Prioritise irrigating the eyes and face. **Call 999/112.**

Poisoning

A poison can be described as any substance *(solid, liquid or gas)* that causes damage when it enters the body in sufficient quantity.

A poison can enter the body in 4 ways, it can be:

Ingested	Swallowed.
Inhaled	Breathed in, entering the blood stream very quickly as it passes through the lungs.
Absorbed	Through the skin or eyes.
Injected	Through the skin, directly into tissues or a blood vessel.

A poison can either be:

Corrosive Such as acids, bleach or ammonia.

OR

Non-corrosive Such as tablets, drugs, alcohol, plants or perfume.

Treatment

For a corrosive substance:

- Don't endanger yourself – make sure it's safe to help.
- Dilute the substance or wash it away if possible:
  - Substances on the skin – wash away with water *(see burns)*.
  - Swallowed substances – if the casualty can swallow and does not feel sick – get them to rinse out the mouth then give frequent sips of milk or water.
- **Call 999/112 for emergency help.** Give information about the poison if possible. Take advice from the ambulance operator.
- If the casualty becomes unconscious – open the **Airway** and check for **Breathing**. Resuscitate if necessary using a protective face shield *(page 15)*. If the casualty is breathing, place them in the recovery position, then **call 999/112**.

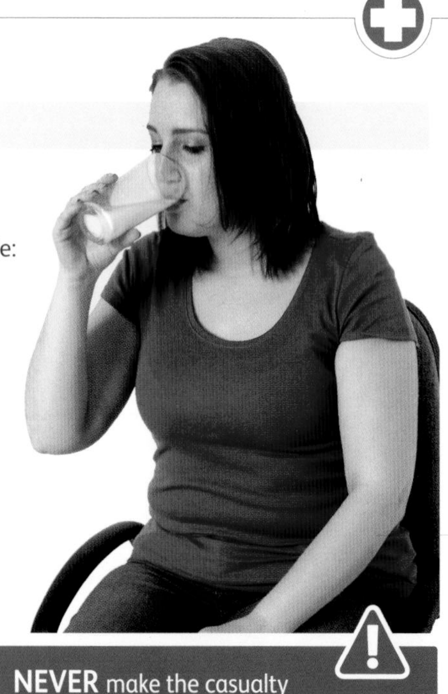

NEVER make the casualty vomit. This may put the airway in danger.

For a non-corrosive substance:

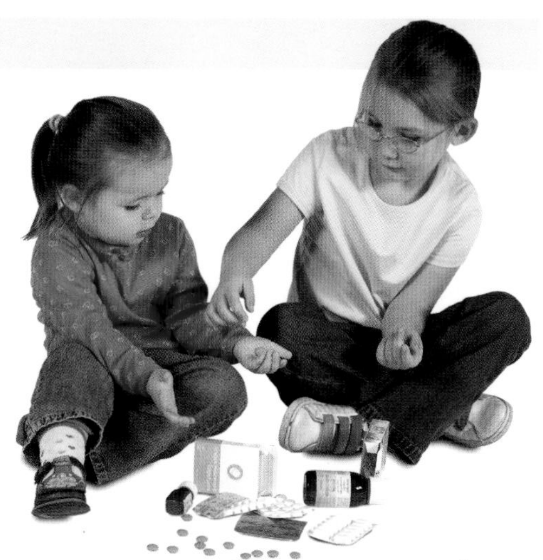

- **Call 999/112 for emergency help**. Give information about the poison if possible. Take advice from the ambulance operator.
- If the casualty becomes unconscious – open the **Airway** and check for **Breathing**. Resuscitate if necessary using a protective face shield *(page 15)*. If the casualty is breathing, place them in the recovery position, then call 999/112.

NOTE: *It helps the paramedics if you:*

- *Pass on containers or other information about the substance.*
- *Find out how much has been taken.*
- *Find out when it was taken.*
- *Keep samples of any vomit for hospital analysis.*

Sources of Information

Specific advice might be found:

- On the container or packaging
- On 'COSHH' safety data sheets
- From an NHS helpline *(e.g. 111)*
- From the ambulance service

Inhalation of smoke, fumes or other substances:

- Move the casualty into fresh air if possible.
- Check **Airway** and **Breathing** *(page 10)* and resuscitate if necessary.
- If the casualty is unconscious – place them in the recovery position *(page 17)*.
- **Call 999/112 for emergency help.**
- If the casualty is conscious and has difficulty breathing, an upright position may help.
- Check for and treat any burns.
- Carefully monitor **Airway** and **Breathing** and resuscitate if necessary.

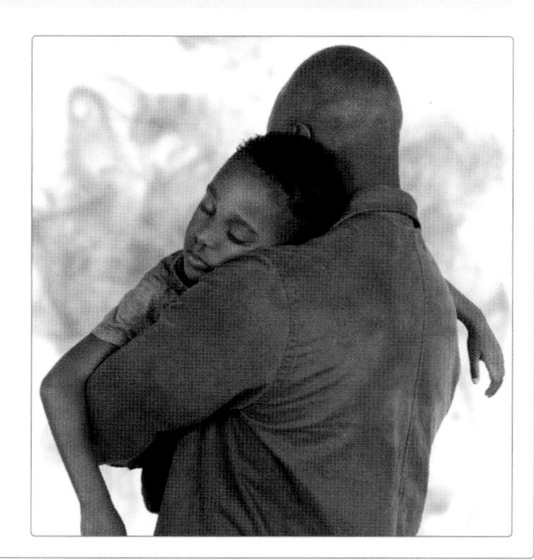

Asthma

An asthma attack is a reaction in the lungs, triggered by such things as dust, pollen, tobacco smoke, exercise, stress or infection.

Muscles surrounding the tiny wind pipes in the lungs go into spasm and constrict, making it very difficult for the casualty to breathe.

Most asthma patients carry medication in the form of an inhaler. Ask the casualty, but usually the blue inhaler is for 'emergency' use, opening the wind pipes to relieve the condition.

An asthma attack is a traumatic experience for the casualty, so reassurance and a calm approach from the first aider is essential.

Normal airway

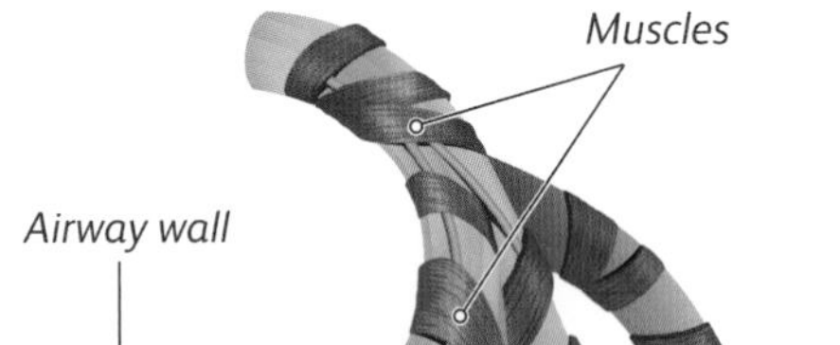

Airway during asthma attack

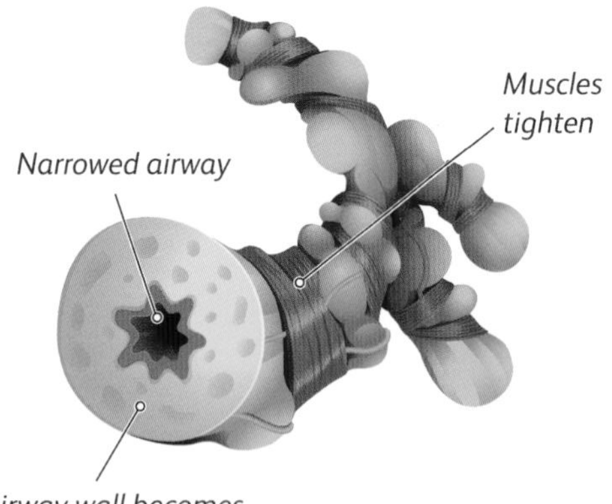

Recognition

- Difficulty breathing and speaking *(has to take a breath mid-sentence)*.
- Wheezy breath sounds originating from the lungs.
- Coughing a lot, or the feeling of a 'tight' chest.
- Pale, clammy skin *(or pale skin inside the lips)* – with grey or blue lips if the attack is severe.
- Use of muscles in the neck and upper chest when breathing.
- Exhaustion in a severe attack.
- May become unconscious and stop breathing in a prolonged attack.

Treatment

- Help the casualty to sit upright, leaning on a table or chair if necessary.
- The casualty should take one puff of their reliever inhaler *(usually blue)* every 30–60 seconds, for up to 10 puffs. Use a spacer device if available.
- Try to take the casualty's mind off the attack – be calm, reassuring and make light conversation.
- **Call 999/112 for emergency help** if they feel worse at any point, or if they don't feel better after 10 puffs. The '10 puff inhaler routine' can be repeated after a few minutes if the ambulance hasn't arrived yet.
- Cold winter air can make an attack worse so don't take the casualty outside for fresh air!
- Keep the casualty upright – even if they become too weak to sit up on their own. Only lay an asthma attack casualty down if they become deeply unconscious.

"Silence in asthma is not good, it is deadly."

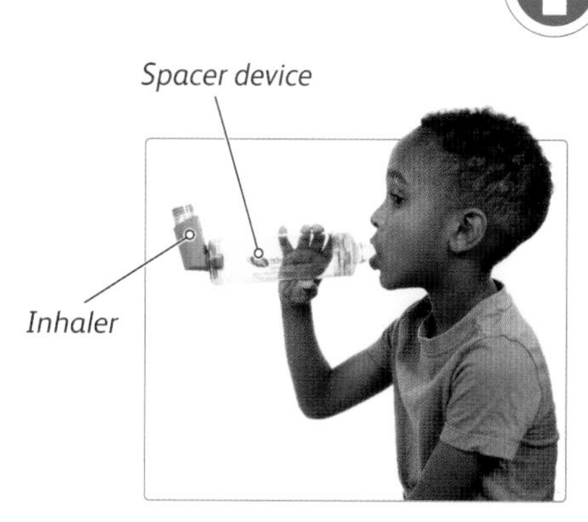

Use a spacer device if available.

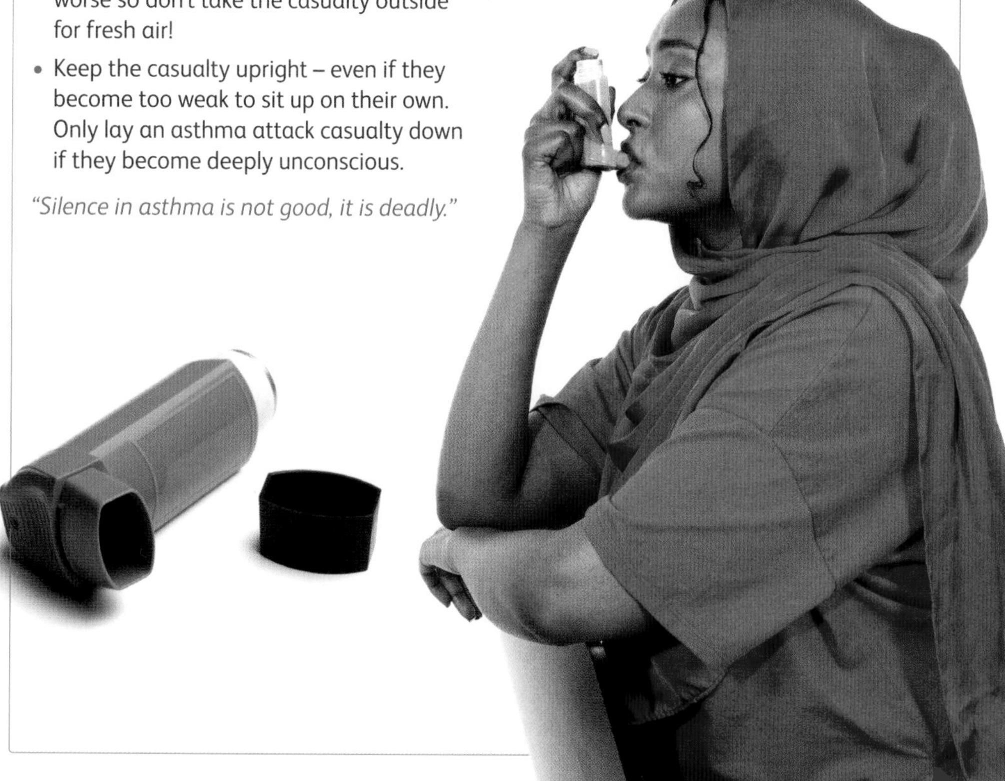

Anaphylaxis

Anaphylaxis is an extremely dangerous allergic reaction. Common triggers are prescribed drugs, insect stings, nuts or seafood.

In anaphylaxis, a chemical called ***histamine*** is over-produced, causing one or more life-threatening **Airway, Breathing** or **Circulation** problems.

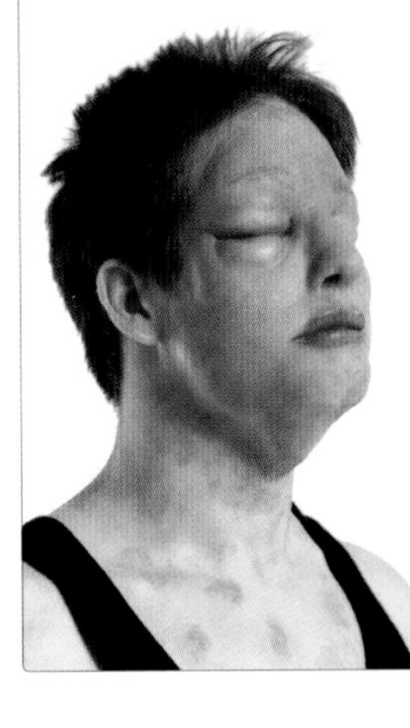

Recognition

- Blotchy skin rash or flushing *(not always present)*.
- A rapid onset and rapid progression of one *(or more)* life-threatening **Airway**, **Breathing** or **Circulation** problems:

  Airway: Blood capillaries can 'leak' causing swelling and blockage. Look out for swelling of the tongue, lips, throat or a feeling of the throat 'closing up'.

  Breathing: Wind-pipes can constrict just like asthma *(page 48)*.

  Circulation: Blood vessels can dilate to **3 times** their usual size, causing a life-threatening fall in blood pressure. Look out for dizziness, fainting, pale skin *(or pale skin inside the lips)* and fast pulse.

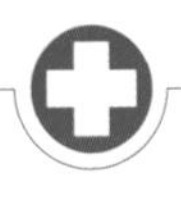

Treatment

- **Call 999/112 for emergency help.**
- Lay the casualty down in a comfortable position. If they feel light-headed or faint – DO NOT sit them up. Raise the legs if necessary.
- If the casualty has Airway or Breathing problems **only**, they may prefer to sit up; but take extreme care – if they feel light-headed or faint, lay them down immediately.
- The casualty may carry an auto-injector of adrenaline. This can save their life if it's given promptly. The casualty should be able to inject this on their own but, if necessary, assist them to use it.
- If the casualty becomes unconscious – check **Airway** and **Breathing** *(page 10)* and resuscitate if necessary.
- The dose of adrenaline can be repeated after 5 minute intervals if there is no improvement or symptoms return.

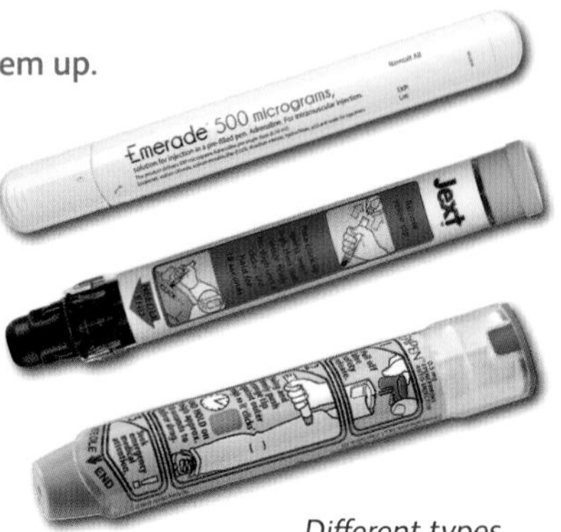

Different types of adrenaline auto-injectors.

Angina and Heart Attack

Angina

Angina is a condition usually caused by the build up of a 'cholesterol plaque' on the inner lining of a coronary artery. Cholesterol is a fatty chemical, which is part of the outer lining of cells in the body. A cholesterol plaque is a hard, thick substance caused by deposits of cholesterol on the artery wall. Over time, the build up of the plaque causes narrowing and hardening of the artery.

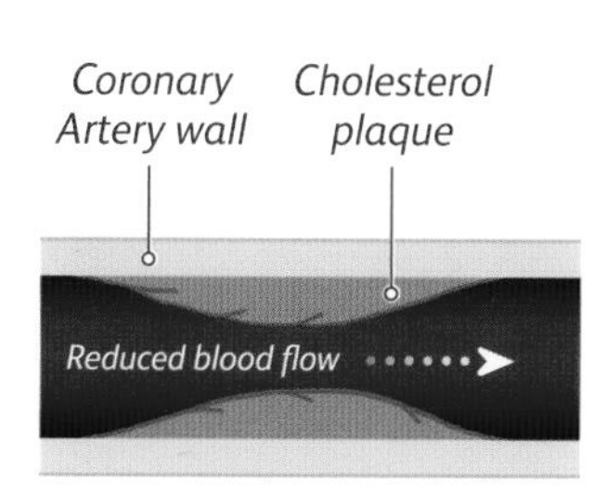

Angina.

During exercise or excitement, the heart needs more oxygen, but the narrowed coronary artery cannot increase the blood supply to meet this demand. As a result an area of the heart will suffer from a lack of oxygen. The casualty usually feels pain in the chest *(amongst other symptoms)* as a result.

Typically an angina attack occurs with exertion and subsides with rest. If the narrowing of the artery reaches a critical level, angina at rest *(called 'unstable angina')* may result. A casualty with unstable angina has a high risk of suffering a heart attack in the near future.

Heart attack

A heart attack is often caused when the surface of a cholesterol plaque in a coronary artery ruptures and the contents leak out.

This leads to the formation of a blood clot, which completely blocks the artery resulting in the **death of an area of the heart muscle**.

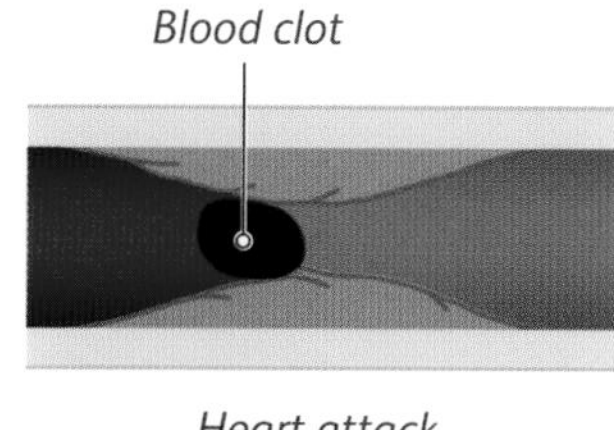

Heart attack.

Unlike angina, the death of the heart muscle from a heart attack is permanent and will not be relieved by rest.

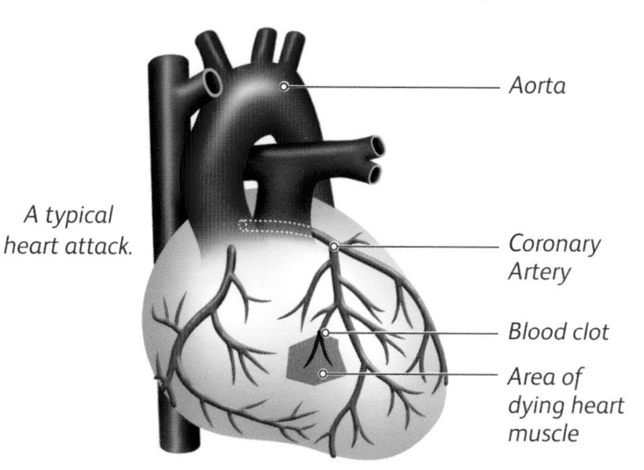

A typical heart attack.

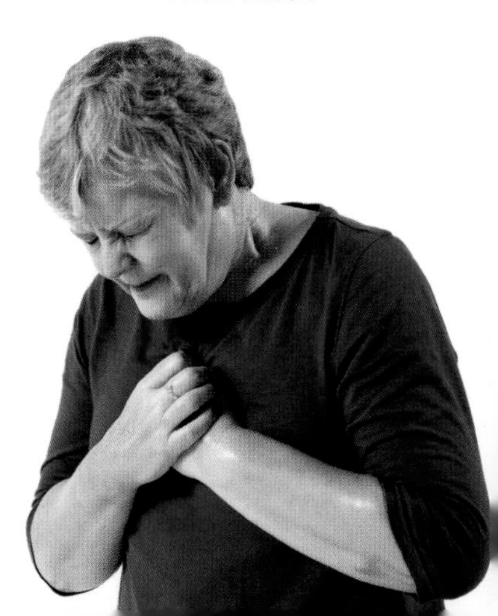

Recognition of angina and heart attack

It should be remembered that every heart attack is different. Only a few of the signs and symptoms may be present, indeed up to a quarter of heart attacks suffered are 'silent' without any chest pain. A silent heart attack is more likely to occur in diabetic patients and the elderly.

	Angina	Heart attack
Onset	Sudden, usually during exertion, stress or extreme weather.	Sudden, can occur at rest.
Pain	'Vice-like' squashing pain, often described as 'dull', 'tightness' or 'pressure' on the chest. Can be mistaken for indigestion.	'Vice-like' squashing pain, often described as 'dull', 'tightness' or 'pressure' on the chest. Can be mistaken for indigestion.
Location of pain	Central chest area. Can radiate into either arm *(more commonly the left)*, the neck, jaw, back, or shoulders.	Central chest area. Can radiate into either arm *(more commonly the left)*, the neck, jaw, back, or shoulders.
Duration	Usually lasts 3 to 8 minutes rarely longer.	Usually lasts longer than 30 minutes.
Skin	Pale skin or pale skin inside the lips.	Pale, grey skin or pale skin inside the lips. May sweat profusely.
Pulse	Variable, depending on which area has a lack of oxygen. Often becomes irregular, missing beats.	Variable, depending on which area has a lack of oxygen. Often becomes irregular, missing beats.
Other signs and symptoms	Shortness of breath, weakness, anxiety.	Shortness of breath, dizziness, nausea, vomiting. Sense of 'impending doom'.
Factors giving relief	Resting, reducing stress, taking 'G.T.N.' medication.	'G.T.N.' medication may give partial or no relief.

Treatment of angina and heart attack

- Sit the casualty down and make them comfortable. Do not allow them to walk around.
- Allow the casualty to take their own glyceryl tri-nitrate *(G.T.N.)* medication if they have it.
- Reassure the casualty. Remove any cause of stress or anxiety if possible.

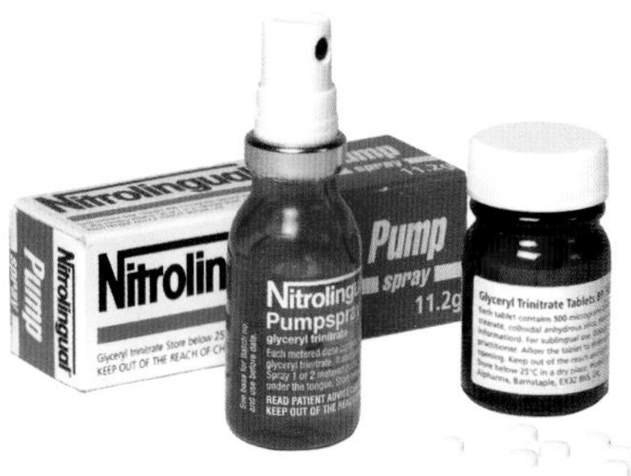

Typical G.T.N. medication that an angina patient may carry.

If you suspect heart attack:

- Bring the nearest AED to the scene as a precaution if available *(only to use if the casualty becomes unconscious and is not breathing normally)*.
- If the casualty is not allergic/sensitive to aspirin and older than 16, allowing them to **chew** an aspirin tablet **slowly** may help to limit the extent of damage to the heart.

  NOTE: *Aspirin reduces the clotting ability of the blood. Chewing the tablet makes it work faster. A 150mg or 300mg chewable or soluble aspirin is ideal.*

- Monitor pulse and breathing. If the casualty becomes unconscious, this usually means the heart has stopped altogether! Be prepared to start CPR and use the AED if needed.

Call 999/112 for emergency help immediately if:

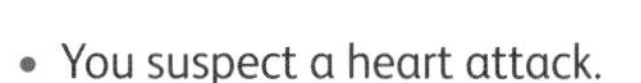

- You suspect a heart attack.
- The casualty has not been diagnosed as having angina.
- The symptoms are different, or worse than the casualty's normal angina attacks.
- Angina pain is not relieved by the casualty's medication and rest after 15 minutes.
- Angina pain has come on whilst the casualty is at rest or it has woken them from their sleep.
- You are in any doubt.

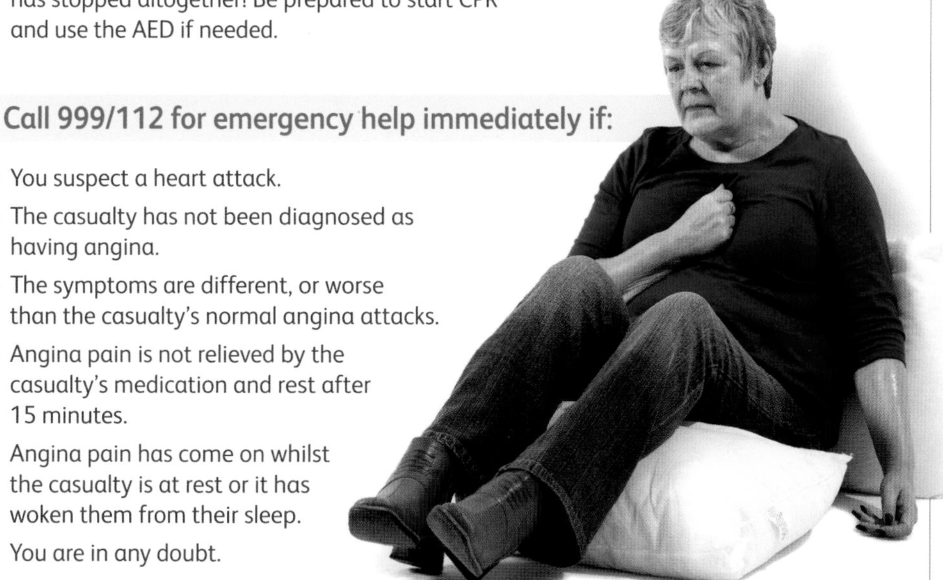

Stroke

There are two types of stroke. The most common is caused by a blood clot, blocking a blood vessel supplying part of the brain. The other is caused if a blood vessel in the brain ruptures, resulting in an area of the brain being 'squashed' by the pressure of the blood.

In either type of stroke, the signs and symptoms are very similar and an area of brain will die. A stroke can happen to a person of any age.

A stroke is a medical emergency. An urgent scan in hospital is required to find out the cause of the stroke, so that the correct treatment can be given quickly. The speed of treatment can have a dramatic impact on the casualty's recovery, but unfortunately it is often delayed because helpers fail to call 999.

Recognition

If you suspect stroke you should carry out the '**FAST**' test:

F **Facial Weakness**
can the person smile? Has their mouth or eye drooped?

A **Arm Weakness**
can the person keep both arms raised?

S **Speech Problems**
can the person speak clearly and understand what you say?

T **Time to call 999/112**
if they fail **any** test, because stroke is a medical emergency.

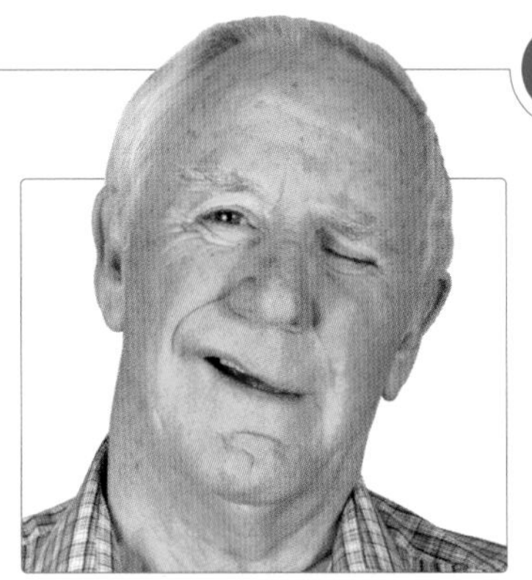

Ask the casualty to smile.

Other red flag symptoms:

- **Balance:** sudden loss of balance, trouble walking, dizziness or loss of coordination.
- **Eyes:** sudden vision loss, double vision or partial loss of vision in one or both eyes.
- Sudden severe headache, nausea or vomiting.

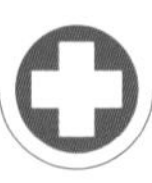

Treatment

- Maintain **Airway** and **Breathing** *(page 10)*.
- **Call 999/112 for emergency help.**
- Place an unconscious casualty in the recovery position *(page 17)*.
- Lay the conscious casualty down, with head and shoulders raised.
- Reassure the casualty – do not assume that they don't understand.
- Monitor and record breathing, pulse and levels of response.

Diabetes

In simple terms, diabetes is related to not producing enough of a hormone called insulin.

Insulin works in the body to 'burn off' the sugars that we eat. Some diabetics have such a lack of insulin that they have to inject insulin to keep their sugar levels down. This type of diabetic is called 'insulin dependent'.

Insulin dependent diabetics have to eat the right amount of sugar to match the insulin injected. If they don't eat enough sugar *(e.g. missing a meal)*, the insulin injection still burns off the small amount of sugar left, so sugar levels can drop dangerously low.

Low blood sugar is dangerous because brain cells, unlike other cells in the body, only use glucose *(sugar)* as their energy supply, so the brain is literally starved.

Recognition of low blood sugar

- Sudden onset and gets worse quickly.
- Strange, uncharacteristic, uncooperative, possibly violent behaviour. Can be mistaken for 'drunkenness'.
- Pale skin *(or pale skin inside the lips)*, cold and sweaty.
- Unconsciousness if not treated.
- Shallow, rapid breathing. Fast pulse.
- The casualty may have an insulin pen, glucose gel, a warning card, or a medic-alert bracelet or necklace.

NEVER give food or drink if the casualty is unconscious.

There is about 20g of glucose in:

- 200ml of pure fruit juice
- 200ml fizzy drink *(not diet)**
- 4 teaspoons of sugar in water
- 4 jelly babies

*Check labels for exact carbohydrate content

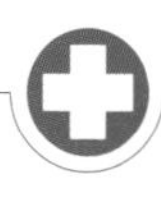

Treatment of low blood sugar

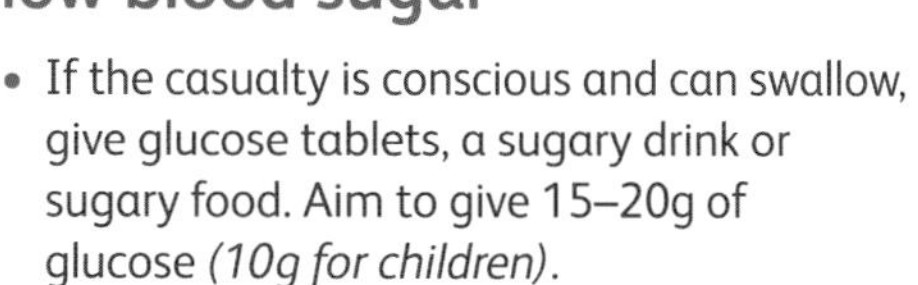

- If the casualty is conscious and can swallow, give glucose tablets, a sugary drink or sugary food. Aim to give 15–20g of glucose *(10g for children)*.
- If they respond to treatment quickly, give more food or drink. Stay with them until they know what month it is.
- If they are unmanageable or do not respond to treatment within 15 minutes **call 999/112 for emergency help**.
- Consider if there is another cause for the casualty's symptoms.
- **If the casualty becomes unconscious**, maintain **Airway** and **Breathing** *(page 10)*, place them in the recovery position *(page 17)* and **call 999/112 for emergency help**.

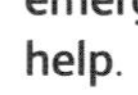

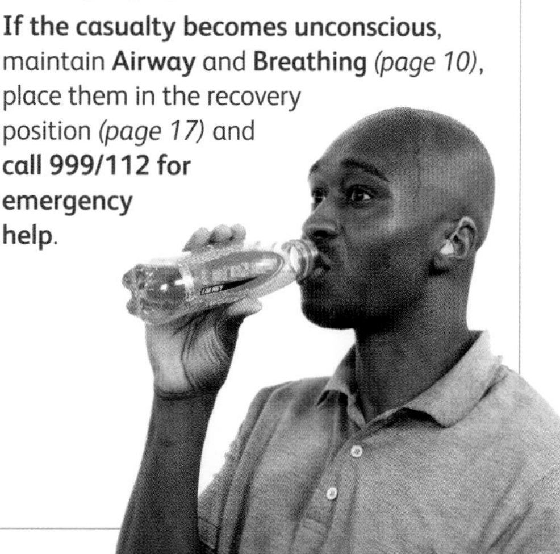

Choking – baby *(under 1 year)*

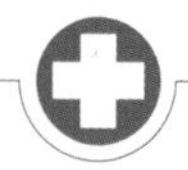

The baby may attempt to cough. If the choking is only mild, this will clear the obstruction – the baby may cry and should now be able to breathe effectively.

If coughing is absent or ineffective:

1 Back blows

- **Shout for help** – ask someone to **call 999/112** or call on a speaker-phone if you can do this **at the same time** as giving treatment.
- Sit or kneel and lay the baby over your lap, face down, head lowest, supporting the head *(see picture)*.
- Give up to 5 sharp blows between the shoulder blades with the heel of your hand. The aim is to relieve the choking with each blow rather than to give all 5.

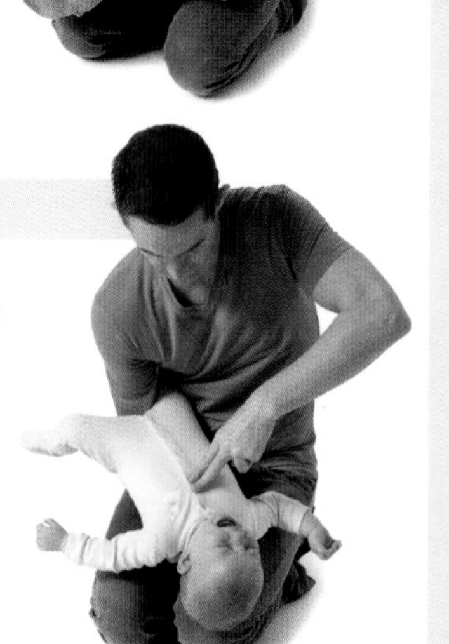

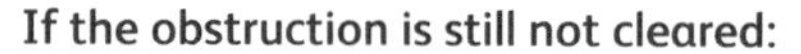

If the obstruction is still not cleared:

2 Chest thrusts

- Turn the baby chest uppermost *(lay them on your arm)*. Support the head and lower it below the level of the chest.
- Use 2 fingers to give up to 5 chest thrusts. These are similar to chest compressions but sharper in nature and delivered at a slower rate. The aim is to relieve the choking with each thrust rather than to give all 5.

NEVER perform abdominal thrusts on a baby.

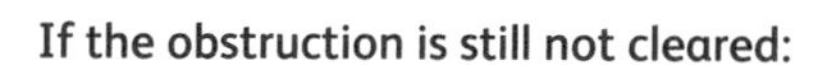

If the obstruction is still not cleared:

3 Repeat steps 1 and 2

- Keep repeating steps 1 and 2.
- If the treatment seems ineffective, make sure someone has **called 999/112 for emergency help**.

If the baby becomes unconscious – START CPR *(pages 10–14)*.

NOTE: *information on when to seek medical attention is on page 20.*

Notes

Hyperthimia - To hot -
Hypothirmia - To cold -

Notes

Notes

Notes

Notes

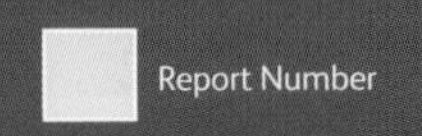

Report Number

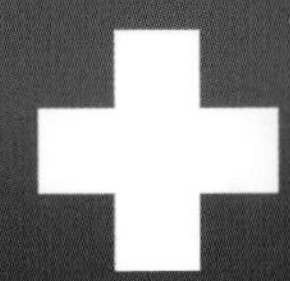

ACCIDENT RECORD

1 About the person who had the accident

Name

Address

Postcode

Occupation

2 About you, the person filling in this record

▼ If you did not have the accident write your address and occupation.

Name

Address

Postcode

Occupation

3 About the accident *Continue on the back of this form if you need to*

▼ Say when it happened. Date / / Time

▼ Say where it happened. State which room or place.

▼ Say how the accident happened. Give the cause if you can.

▼ If the person who had the accident suffered an injury, say what it was.

▼ Please sign the record and date it.

Signature Date / /

4 For the employee only

☐ By ticking this box I give my consent to my employer to disclose my personal information and details of the accident which appear on this form to safety representatives and representatives of employee safety for them to carry out the health and safety functions given to them by law.

Signature Date / /

5 For the employer only

Complete this box if the accident is reportable under the Reporting of injuries, Diseases and Dangerous Occurrences Regulations (RIDDOR).
To report, go to **http://www.hse.gov.uk/riddor/report.htm**

How was it reported?

Signature Date reported / /

Resuscitation flow chart

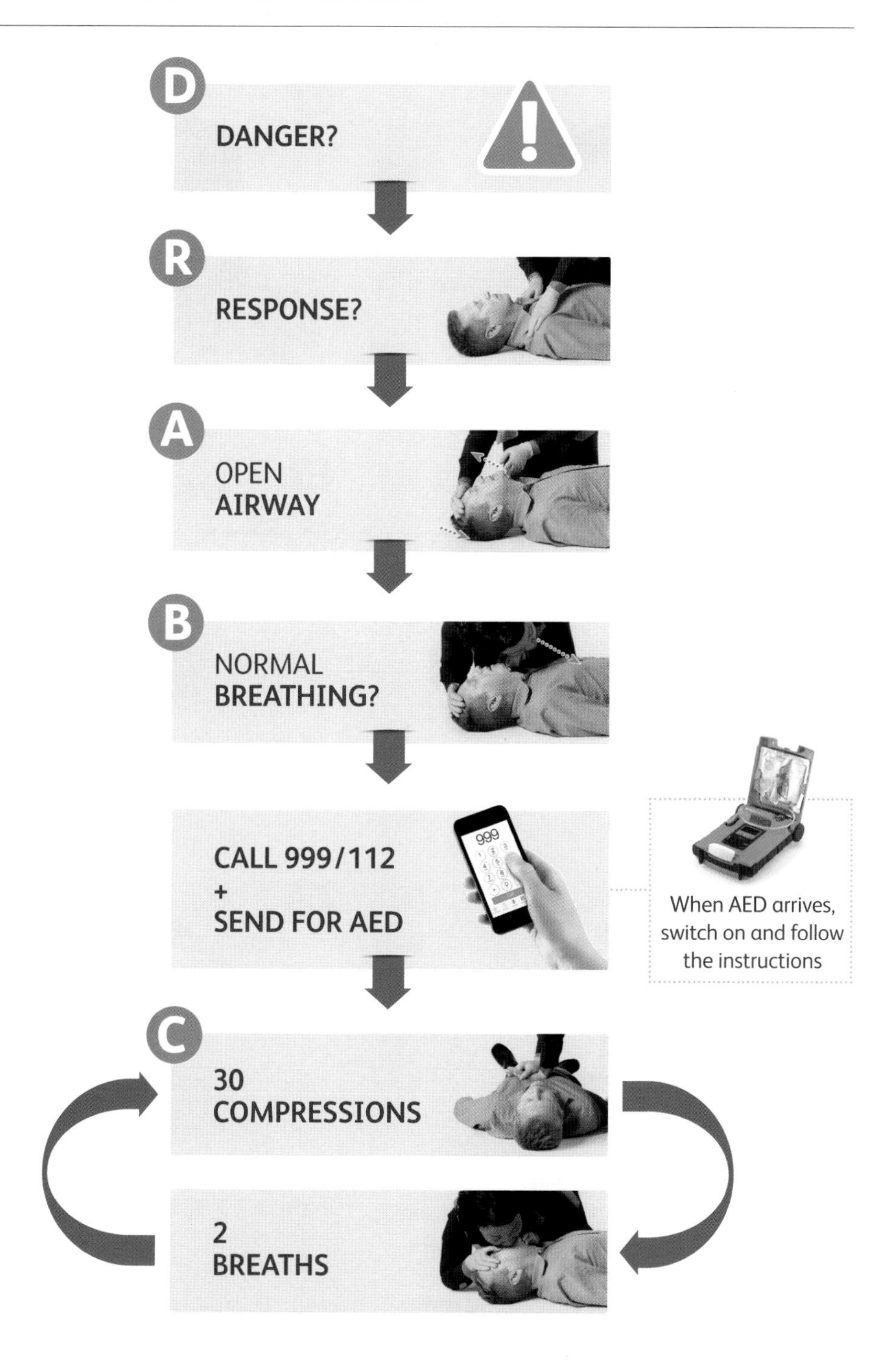

COVID-19 CPR adaptations

1

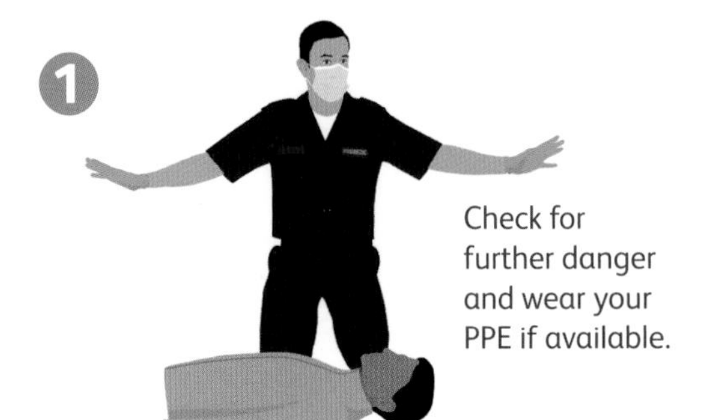

Check for further danger and wear your PPE if available.

2

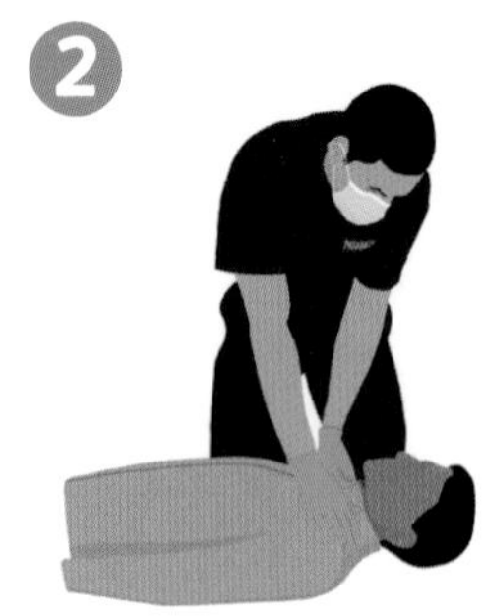

At arms length, check for response by gently shaking the shoulders and shout loudly.

At arms length, check for normal breathing for no longer than 10 seconds. You can place your hand on the abdomen, just below the ribs to check for movement.

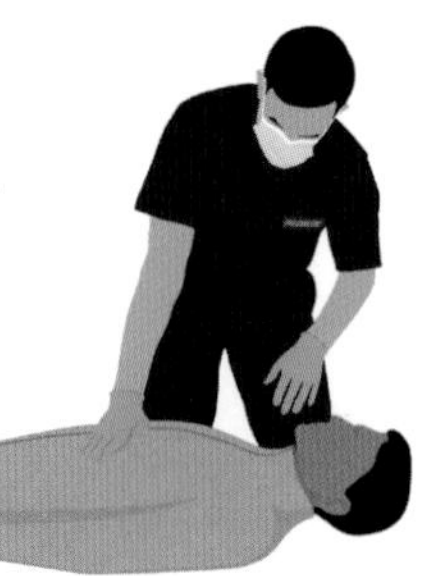

DO NOT place your face near the casualty's mouth.

DO NOT tip the head back to open the airway.

4

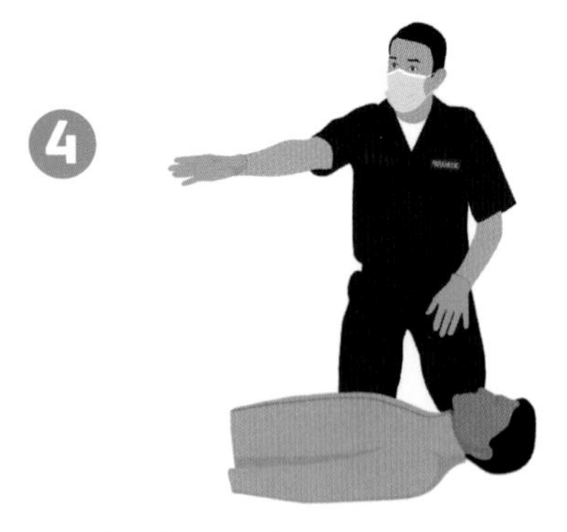

Call 999 or 112 and send for a defibrillator if available.

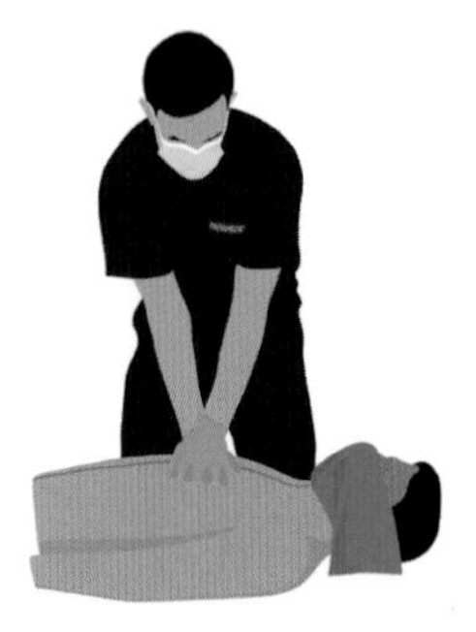

Unresponsive and not breathing normally?

Place some material over the casualty's mouth and nose *(e.g. tea towel)*, then give **continuous chest compressions** at a rate of about 2 per second and 5–6cm deep. Press 'hard and fast'.

6

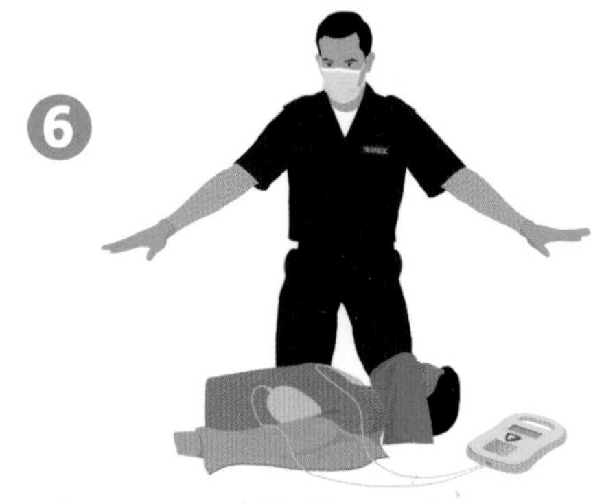

As soon as a defibrillator arrives, switch it on and follow the instructions. This is completely safe to use even with COVID-19.